Cranial Nerve Stimulation in Otolaryngology

Editors

JAMES G. NAPLES
MICHAEL J. RUCKENSTEIN

OTOLARYNGOLOGIC CLINICS OF NORTH AMERICA

www.oto.theclinics.com

Consulting Editor
SUJANA S. CHANDRASEKHAR

February 2020 • Volume 53 • Number 1

ELSEVIER

1600 John F. Kennedy Boulevard • Suite 1800 • Philadelphia, Pennsylvania, 19103-2899

http://www.oto.theclinics.com

OTOLARYNGOLOGIC CLINICS OF NORTH AMERICA Volume 53, Number 1
February 2020 ISSN 0030-6665, ISBN-13: 978-0-323-71056-5

Editor: Stacy Eastman
Developmental Editor: Laura Fisher

Otolaryngologic Clinics of North America (ISSN 0030-6665) is published bimonthly by Elsevier, Inc., 360 Park Avenue South, New York, NY 10010-1710. Months of issue are February, April, June, August, October, and December. Business and Editorial Offices: 1600 John F. Kennedy Blvd., Suite 1800, Philadelphia, PA 19103-2899. Customer Service Office: 6277 Sea Harbor Drive, Orlando, FL 32887-4800. Periodicals postage paid at New York, NY and additional mailing offices. Subscription prices are $424.00 per year (US individuals), $947.00 per year (US institutions), $100.00 per year (US & Canadian student/resident), $548.00 per year (Canadian individuals), $1200.00 per year (Canadian institutions), $592.00 per year (international individuals), $1200.00 per year (international institutions), $270.00 per year (international student/resident). Foreign air speed delivery is included in all *Clinics*' subscription prices. All prices are subject to change without notice. **POSTMASTER:** Send address changes to *Otolaryngologic Clinics of North America*, Elsevier Health Sciences Division, Subscription Customer Service, 3251 Riverport Lane, Maryland Heights, MO 63043. **Telephone: 1-800-654-2452 (U.S. and Canada); 314-447-8871 (outside U.S. and Canada). Fax: 314-447-8029. E-mail: journalscustomerservice-usa@elsevier.com (for print support); journalsonlinesupport-usa@elsevier.com (for online support).**

Reprints. For copies of 100 or more of articles in this publication, please contact the Commercial Reprints Department, Elsevier Inc., 360 Park Avenue South, New York, NY 10010-1710. Tel.: 212-633-3874; Fax: 212-633-3820; E-mail: reprints@elsevier.com.

Otolaryngologic Clinics of North America is also published in Spanish by McGraw-Hill Interamericana Editores S.A., P.O. Box 5-237, 06500 Mexico D.F., Mexico.

Otolaryngologic Clinics of North America is covered in *MEDLINE/PubMed (Index Medicus)*, *Current Contents/Clinical Medicine*, *Excerpta Medica*, *BIOSIS*, *Science Citation Index*, and *ISI/BIOMED*.

Contributors

CONSULTING EDITOR

SUJANA S. CHANDRASEKHAR, MD, FACS, FAAOHNS
Past President, American Academy of Otolaryngology–Head and Neck Surgery,
Secretary-Treasurer, American Otological Society, Partner, ENT & Allergy Associates,
LLP, Clinical Professor, Department of Otolaryngology–Head and Neck Surgery, Zucker
School of Medicine at Hofstra-Northwell, Hempstead, New York, USA; Clinical Associate
Professor, Department of Otolaryngology–Head and Neck Surgery, Icahn School of
Medicine at Mount Sinai, New York, New York, USA

EDITORS

JAMES G. NAPLES, MD
Division of Otolaryngology, Beth Israel Deaconess Medical Center, Harvard Medical
School, Boston, Massachusetts, USA

MICHAEL J. RUCKENSTEIN, MD
Department of Otorhinolaryngology–Head and Neck Surgery, University of Pennsylvania
Health System, Philadelphia, Pennsylvania, USA

AUTHORS

KSENIA A. AARON, MD
Department of Otolaryngology–Head and Neck Surgery, Stanford University School of
Medicine, Stanford, California, USA

M. CHRISTIAN BROWN, PhD
Massachusetts Eye and Ear Infirmary, Harvard Medical School, Boston, Massachusetts,
USA

DANIEL H. COELHO, MD
Professor, Department of Otolaryngology–Head and Neck Surgery, Virginia
Commonwealth University School of Medicine, Richmond, Virginia, USA

NICHOLAS L. DEEP, MD
Neurotology Fellow, Department of Otolaryngology-Head and Neck Surgery, NYU
Langone Health, New York, New York, USA

NILS GUINAND, MD, PhD
Division of Otorhinolaryngology and Head and Neck Surgery, Department of Clinical
Neurosciences, Geneva University Hospitals, Geneva, Switzerland

SVEN OVE HANSSON, PhD
Professor, Division of Philosophy, Royal Institute of Technology (KTH), Stockholm,
Sweden; Department of Learning, Informatics, Management and Ethics, Karolinska
Institutet, Sweden

ERIC H. HOLBROOK, MD
Associate Professor, Department of Otolaryngology–Head and Neck Surgery, Massachusetts Eye and Ear Infirmary, Harvard Medical School, Boston, Massachusetts, USA

HERMANUS KINGMA, PhD
Department of Otorhinolaryngology–Head and Neck Surgery, School for Mental Health and Neuroscience, Faculty of Health Medicine and Life Sciences, Maastricht University Medical Center, Maastricht, The Netherlands

GAVRIEL D. KOHLBERG, MD
Assistant Professor of Otology and Neurotology, Department of Otolaryngology– Head and Neck Surgery, University of Washington School of Medicine, Seattle, Washington, USA

ELLIOTT D. KOZIN, MD
Department of Otolaryngology, Massachusetts Eye and Ear Infirmary, and Harvard Medical School, Boston, Massachusetts, USA

DANIEL J. LEE, MD
Department of Otolaryngology, Massachusetts Eye and Ear Infirmary, Harvard Medical School, Boston, Massachusetts, USA

ALBERT C. MUDRY, MD, PhD
Department of Otolaryngology–Head and Neck Surgery, Stanford University School of Medicine, Stanford, California, USA

ANDREAS H. MUELLER, MD
Chair, Otorhinolaryngology, SRH Wald-Klinikum, Gera, Germany

JAMES G. NAPLES, MD
Division of Otolaryngology, Beth Israel Deaconess Medical Center, Harvard Medical School, Boston, Massachusetts, USA

KWAKU K. OHEMENG, BS
Department of Surgery, Division of Otolaryngology–Head and Neck Surgery, UConn School of Medicine, UConn Health, Farmington, Connecticut, USA

KOUROSH PARHAM, MD, PhD
Associate Professor, Department of Surgery, Division of Otolaryngology–Head and Neck Surgery, UConn School of Medicine, UConn Health, Farmington, Connecticut, USA

ANGÉLICA PÉREZ FORNOS, PhD
Division of Otorhinolaryngology and Head and Neck Surgery, Department of Clinical Neurosciences, Geneva University Hospitals, Geneva, Switzerland

ALIDA ANNECHIEN POSTMA, MD, PhD
Department of Radiology and Nuclear Medicine, School for Mental Health and Neuroscience, Faculty of Health Medicine and Life Sciences, Maastricht University Medical Center, Maastricht, The Netherlands

CLAUS POTOTSCHNIG, MD
Consultant, Otorhinolaryngology, Innsbruck University Hospital, Innsbruck, Austria

AHAD A. QURESHI, MD
Department of Otolaryngology, Massachusetts Eye and Ear Infirmary, Harvard Medical School, Boston, Massachusetts, USA

J. THOMAS ROLAND Jr, MD
Mendik Foundation Chairman, Professor of Otolaryngology and Neurosurgery, Department of Otolaryngology-Head and Neck Surgery, NYU Langone Health, New York, New York, USA

MICHAEL J. RUCKENSTEIN, MD
Department of Otorhinolaryngology–Head and Neck Surgery, University of Pennsylvania Health System, Philadelphia, Pennsylvania, USA

RAVI N. SAMY, MD, FACS
Professor and Chief, Division of Otology/Neurotology, Program Director, Neurotology Fellowship, Department of Otolaryngology–Head and Neck Surgery, University of Cincinnati College of Medicine, Neurosensory Disorders Center at University of Cincinnati Gardner Neuroscience Institute, Cincinnati Children's Hospital Medical Center, Cincinnati, Ohio, USA

JEFFREY D. SHARON, MD
Department of Otolaryngology–Head and Neck Surgery, University of California San Francisco, San Francisco, California, USA

KONSTANTINA M. STANKOVIC, MD, PhD
Massachusetts Eye and Ear Infirmary, Harvard Medical School, Boston, Massachusetts, USA

JOOST JOHANNES ANTONIUS STULTIENS, MD
Department of Otorhinolaryngology–Head and Neck Surgery, School for Mental Health and Neuroscience, Faculty of Health Medicine and Life Sciences, Maastricht University Medical Center, Maastricht, The Netherlands

ERICA R. THALER, MD
Professor of Otorhinolaryngology: Head and Neck Surgery, Department of Otorhinolaryngology, Hospital of the University of Pennsylvania, Philadelphia, Pennsylvania, USA

RAYMOND VAN DE BERG, MD, PhD
Department of Otorhinolaryngology–Head and Neck Surgery, School for Mental Health and Neuroscience, Faculty of Health Medicine and Life Sciences, Maastricht University Medical Center, Maastricht, The Netherlands

HEATHER M. WEINREICH, MD, MPH
Department of Otolaryngology–Head and Neck Surgery, University of Illinois–Chicago, Chicago, Illinois, USA

JOHANNA L. WICKEMEYER, MD
Department of Otolaryngology–Head and Neck Surgery, University of Illinois–Chicago, Chicago, Illinois, USA

JASON L. YU, MD
Fellow, Division of Sleep Medicine, Hospital of the University of Pennsylvania, Philadelphia, Pennsylvania, USA

ANGELA ZHU, MPhil
Department of Otolaryngology, Massachusetts Eye and Ear Infirmary, Harvard Medical School, Boston, Massachusetts, USA

Contents

> This article aims to clearly understand the historical development of cranial nerve–implanted stimulators in otolaryngology. The authors also discuss cranial nerve history; initial theory of the functional concept of animal spirit; electrical nerve impulse theory; first electrical otolaryngology cranial nerve stimulation devices; and the development of implanted stimulators.

> This overview of ethical and social issues pertaining to cranial nerve implants covers informed consent; risk-benefit assessments; security against unauthorized reprogramming or privacy intrusion; explantation; psychological side effects; equity and social distribution, cultural effects, for instance, on the deaf subculture; enhancement; and research ethics.

> Understanding the mechanisms of neural stimulation is necessary to improve the management of sensory disorders. Neurons can be artificially stimulated using electrical current, or with newer stimulation modalities, including optogenetics. Electrical stimulation forms the basis for all neuroprosthetic devices that are used clinically. Off-target stimulation and poor implant performance remain concerns for patients with electrically based neuroprosthetic devices. Optogenetic techniques may improve cranial nerve stimulation strategies used by various neuroprostheses and result in better patient outcomes. This article reviews the fundamentals of neural stimulation and provides an overview of recent major advancements in light-based neuromodulation.

> The current literature on peripheral cranial nerve stimulation for the purpose of achieving therapeutic effects via altering brain activity is reviewed. Vagus nerve stimulation, which is approved for use in refractory epilepsy,

is the most extensively studied cranial nerve stimulator that has direct impact on the central nervous system. Despite the recognized central effects of peripheral cranial nerve stimulation, the mechanism of action for all indications remains incompletely understood. Further research on both mechanisms and indications of central effects of cranial nerve stimulation has the potential to alleviate burden of disease in a large array of conditions.

auditory nerve. They are used in patients who are not cochlear implant candidates. Current criteria for use in the United States are neurofibromatosis type 2 patients 12 years or older undergoing first- or second-side vestibular schwannoma removal. However, there are other nontumor conditions in which patients may benefit from an ABI, such as bilateral cochlear nerve aplasia and severe cochlear malformation not amendable to cochlear implantation. Recent experience with ABI in the pediatric population demonstrates good safety profile and encouraging results.

Recent research has shown promising results for the development of a clinically feasible vestibular implant in the near future. However, correct electrode placement remains a challenge. It was shown that fluoroscopy was able to visualize the semicircular canal ampullae and electrodes, and guide electrode insertion in real time. Ninety-four percent of the 18 electrodes were implanted correctly (<1.5 mm distance to target). The median distances were 0.60 mm, 0.85 mm, and 0.65 mm for the superior, lateral, and posterior semicircular canal, respectively. These findings suggest that fluoroscopy can significantly improve electrode placement during vestibular implantation.

Vagal nerve stimulation (VNS) therapy is a surgical treatment that involves the implantation of a device to electrically stimulate the vagus nerve. It is indicated as an adjunctive treatment of epilepsy that is refractory to antiepileptic medications and for treatment-resistant depression. The exact mechanism by which VNS achieves its effects is not known, but various mechanisms have been proposed, including afferent vagal projections to seizure-generating regions of the brain and desynchronization of hypersynchronized cortical activity. The most common complications of VNS therapy include hoarseness, throat pain/dysphagia, coughing, and shortness of breath.

Electrical stimulation of the recurrent laryngeal nerve is a safe and promising therapeutic approach with the potentiality to overcome the shortcomings of conventional surgical glottal enlargement. Although aberrant or synkinetic reinnervation is commonly considered an unfavorable condition, particularly for recovery of vocal fold movement, its presence is essential to ensure the effective clinical performance of laryngeal pacemakers. Thus, the effective selection of patients who can profit from laryngeal pacemakers implantation demands the implementation of new diagnostic tools based on tests capable of reliably detecting the presence of viable reinnervation on at least one vocal fold.

Hypoglossal nerve stimulation is a novel strategy for the treatment of obstructive sleep apnea (OSA). Its anatomy allows for easy surgical access, and its function as a motor nerve allows for tolerable neurostimulation. It has shown success as a therapy for the treatment of OSA with a greater than 80% success rate. Patients who use the device not only show improvement in symptoms but also tolerate the device well with high rates of adherence to therapy as well as a high majority preferring it over continuous positive airway pressure therapy.

Despite advances in implant hardware, neuroprosthetic devices in otolaryngology have sustained evolutionary rather than revolutionary changes over the past half century. Although electrical stimulation has the capacity for facile activation of neurons and high temporal resolution, it has limited spatial selectivity. Alternative strategies for neuronal stimulation are being investigated to improve spatial resolution. In particular, light-based neuronal stimulation is a viable alternative and complement to electrical stimulation. This article provides a broad overview of light-based neuronal stimulation technologies. Specific examples of active research on light-based prostheses, including cochlear implants, auditory brainstem implants, retinal implants, and facial nerve implants, are reviewed.

OTOLARYNGOLOGIC CLINICS
OF NORTH AMERICA

SERIES OF RELATED INTEREST

Facial Plastic Surgery Clinics
Available at: https://www.facialplastic.theclinics.com/

THE CLINICS ARE AVAILABLE ONLINE!
Access your subscription at:
www.theclinics.com

Foreword

Brain-Nerve-Computer Interfaces in Otolaryngology

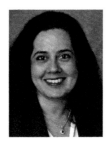

Sujana S. Chandrasekhar, MD, FACS, FAAOHNS
Consulting Editor

Otolaryngologists are concerned with form and function of delicate, intricate structures. Until relatively recently, if a nerve could not be sewn back together or grafted, its function could not be restored. This issue of *Otolaryngologic Clinics of North America*, devoted to Cranial Nerve Stimulation in Otolaryngology and guest edited by Dr Michael Ruckenstein and Dr James Naples, looks at our specialty as it extends past cranial nerve deficits to reach new frontiers of reactivation, of incorporating biomedical technology to the patient experience.

While passive limb prosthetics, for example, have a long history, the most common cranial nerve stimulator used in our field, the cochlear implant (CI), is only decades old. There are plenty of people around who still remember the agitation that was created at the thought of placing an electrode inside a human cochlea on the chance that that person might hear. André Djourno and Charles Eyriès invented the original CI in 1957. Dr William F. House faced stern opposition for over a quarter century while he was developing his CI, the first of which he implanted into a patient in 1961. Before the then-American Academy of Ophthalmology and Otolaryngology endorsed (multichannel) CIs in 1977, doctors and scientists had denounced Dr House, saying the implant would either not work or not work well and calling it a 'cruel hoax to those desperate to hear'.[1] The United States Food and Drug Administration (FDA) first approved cochlear implantation in 1984. Over time and use, CIs have gone from minimal expectations of sound awareness to maximal expectations of normal oral/auditory speech and language development and full restoration in postlingual deafness. Audiometric indications have changed from only profound binaural hearing loss to ears with significant residual hearing. FDA limitations on age have gone from adults only to age 1 year and up, with many implants being performed in infants. Surgical techniques have become streamlined with hearing preservation an achievable goal.

Otolaryngol Clin N Am 53 (2020) xiii–xiv
https://doi.org/10.1016/j.otc.2019.10.001
0030-6665/20/© 2019 Published by Elsevier Inc.

Most importantly, what was an anomaly, a "miracle" if you would, is now considered an obvious choice with expected excellent outcome.

Based on the success of CI, further work has been done looking at cranial nerve stimulation to restore function in other areas of the head and neck. Simultaneous improvements in central nervous system stimulation, such as with deep brain stimulators for severe tremors and peripheral nerve stimulators for spine and extremity disorders, have sped up the development of these self-contained technology-assist devices. In Otolaryngology, we have clinical experience with auditory brainstem implants in neurofibromatosis II or absent cochlear nerves, with hypoglossal nerve stimulators for sleep apnea, and vagal nerve stimulators for debilitating epilepsy. We have seen that stimulation of one cranial nerve target like the tongue base can stimulate improvement in other cranial nerve areas like vestibular function and even vision.[2,3] A future that includes recurrent laryngeal nerve implantation for spasmodic dysphonia and other voice issues, vestibular implantation for absent vestibular function, olfactory nerve stimulators for anosmia, and perhaps other areas of cranial nerve "cross-talk" appears not too distant.

Drs Naples and Ruckenstein have compiled a comprehensive series of articles by thought leaders in different areas of cranial nerve stimulators. Beginning with the history, exploring the ethics, the concepts of electrical and optical modulation, and central effects of stimulators, and continuing on to the different cranial nerves needing stimulators, this issue concludes with what is poised to be the next really big thing, light-based neuronal activation. I hope you enjoy reading this issue and expanding your thinking well outside the box!

Sujana S. Chandrasekhar, MD, FACS, FAAOHNS
Consulting Editor, Otolaryngologic Clinics of North America

Past President, American Academy of Otolaryngology-Head and Neck Surgery
Secretary-Treasurer, American Otological Society Partner, ENT & Allergy Associates,
LLP 18 East 48th Street, 2nd Floor, New York, NY 10017, USA

Clinical Professor, Department of Otolaryngology-Head and Neck Surgery
Zucker School of Medicine at Hofstra-Northwell, Hempstead, NY, USA

Clinical Associate Professor, Department of Otolaryngology-Head and Neck Surgery,
Icahn School of Medicine at Mount Sinai, New York, NY, USA

E-mail address:
ssc@nyotology.com

REFERENCES

1. Eshraghi AA, Nazarian R, Telischi FF, et al. The cochlear implant: historical aspects and future prospects. Anat Rec (Hoboken) 2012;295(11):1967–80. https://doi.org/10.1002/ar.22580.
2. Danilov YP, Tyler ME, Skinner KL, et al. Efficacy of electrotactile vestibular substitution in patients with peripheral and central vestibular loss. J Vestib Res 2007;17(2-3):119–30.
3. Arnoldussen A, Rhode K. Enhanced perception with the BrainPort Vision device. Invest Ophthalmol Vis Sci 2010;51(13):3634.

Preface

The Impact and Evolution of Cranial Nerve Stimulators in Otolaryngology

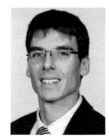 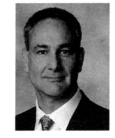

James G. Naples, MD   Michael J. Ruckenstein, MD
Editors

As otolaryngologists, we specialize in the management of various individual organs within an anatomical region. This provides our specialty with a unique opportunity to address a breadth of disorders that are largely related to the special senses and often involve specific input from individual cranial nerves. As such, management of these disorders can be challenging because of the sensitive information being relayed and the complexities involved in cranial nerve signaling. When medical options fail to provide benefit, surgical options become available. However, few surgical options are available for insults that result from cranial nerve dysfunction. This shortcoming is even more apparent because of the impact that sensory and other otolaryngologic disorders have on a patient's quality of life (QOL). Consider the frustration of patients who suffer from disorders that result from cranial nerve dysfunction, such as hearing loss and imbalance, dysphonia and dysphagia, anosmia, or obstructive sleep apnea (OSA).

Fortunately, recent advances in technology have introduced the concept of electrical stimulation of cranial nerves to restore input to various organs within the head and neck. The earliest example is the cochlear implant, which provides direct electrical stimulation to the cochlear nerve. With this electrical stimulator as a prototype, additional cranial nerve stimulators have been developed for use by otolaryngologists. For example, hypoglossal nerve stimulation for OSA is rapidly proving to be a successful option for many patients. Vagal nerve stimulation for various neuropsychiatric disorders is a well-established procedure that some otolaryngologists perform due to their level of comfort with the surgical anatomy of the neck.

The history of the cochlear implant has provided the foundation for our current understanding of cranial nerve stimulators, and we are currently in an era of significant progress to build upon this foundation. At present, the use of hypoglossal nerve

Otolaryngol Clin N Am 53 (2020) xv–xvi
https://doi.org/10.1016/j.otc.2019.09.015
0030-6665/20/© 2019 Published by Elsevier Inc.

stimulators across the country is expanding and will likely soon have a history of its own worthy of discussion. Most exciting, however, is the future of cranial nerve stimulation. Currently, biomedical engineering and early clinical research are being performed to evaluate direct stimulation of the vestibular nerve, olfactory nerve, and recurrent laryngeal nerve. If we use history as our lens for the future, our specialty should anticipate that these significant innovations will soon integrate into our list of treatment options for patients.

This issue of *Otolaryngologic Clinics of North America* tells a story of the history and evolution of cranial nerve stimulators. We review indications for each of the stimulators in clinical use. In addition, we provide details of ethical, technological, medical, and surgical considerations for patients who have these implantable stimulators. Finally, we offer the latest research on the design and role of new cranial nerve stimulators that are certain to be a part of the future of otolaryngology.

Our specialty is responsible for the discovery of many of the early tools necessary to successfully restore deficits that range from sound to sleep through cranial nerve stimulation. Restoration of speech, swallow, smell, and balance is soon to follow. As a specialty, we are pioneering a concept that integrates the complexities of biomedical engineering, surgery, and improving patient QOL. We hope that this issue will provide practical information for the otolaryngologist in understanding cranial nerve stimulation and managing patients with these implants, while also offering expectations for future management options of challenging otolaryngologic disorders with cranial nerve stimulators.

James G. Naples, MD
Beth Israel Deaconess Medical Center
Harvard Medical School
Otolaryngology-Head and Neck Surgery
110 Francis Street, Suite E
Boston, MA 02215, USA

Michael J. Ruckenstein, MD
University of Pennsylvania Health System
Department of Otorhinolaryngology–Head and Neck Surgery
3400 Spruce Street, 5 Silverstein
Philadelphia, PA 19104, USA

E-mail addresses:
Jnaples513@gmail.com (J.G. Naples)
Michael.ruckenstein@uphs.upenn.edu (M.J. Ruckenstein)

History of Cranial Nerve–Implanted Stimulators in Otolaryngology

Ksenia A. Aaron, MD*, Albert C. Mudry, MD, PhD[1]

KEYWORDS

- Cranial nerve • Implant • Stimulators • Otolaryngology

KEY POINTS

- To clearly understand the historical development of cranial nerve–implanted stimulators in otolaryngology.
- To describe cranial nerve history; initial theory of the functional concept of animal spirit; electrical nerve impulse theory; and first electrical otolaryngology cranial nerve stimulation devices.
- To present recent development of implanted stimulators.

INTRODUCTION

Described since Antiquity, the cranial nerves found their actual numbering classification and arrangement in 1778, by Soemmerring,[1] who repertorized them in 12 pairs.[2] Seven of them, more or less, concern the specialty of Otolaryngology, Head and Neck Surgery: olfactory nerve I, trigeminal nerve V, facial nerve VII, cochleovestibular nerve VIII, glossopharyngeal nerve IX, vagus nerve X, and hypoglossal nerve XII. These nerves are associated with 3 different types of peripheral receptors: sensory for nerves I (olfaction), VII, IX, X (taste), and VIII (audition); motors for VII, X, and XII; and pain and insensibility (anesthesia) for V. Since the mid twentieth century, various devices, external and implanted, were produced to directly stimulate the function of these otolaryngology cranial nerves (OCN), the most well known and successful one being the cochlear implant (CI).

The aim of this research is to study the history and development of cranial nerve–implanted stimulators in otolaryngology. An extensive review of the literature was conducted from secondary references to original ones since antiquity and thus in different languages. Interestingly, as large were studies of stimulation of hearing, as less were

Department of Otolaryngology–Head and Neck Surgery, Stanford University School of Medicine, Stanford, CA, USA
[1] Present address: 801 Welch Road, Palo Alto, CA 94305.
* Corresponding author. 801 Welch Road, Palo Alto, CA 94305.
E-mail address: kaaron@stanford.edu

of smell and taste! As it is a quite extensive domain, only some specific points were extracted to clarify the subject.

To clearly understand the historical development of OCN-implanted stimulators, different steps must be presented: first description of cranial nerves; the initial theory of the functional concept of animal spirit; the original attempts to stimulate this animal spirit, that is, functional stimulation; the introduction and understanding of electrical nerve impulse theory; the first electrical OCN stimulation devices; and the development of OCN-implanted stimulators.

FIRST DESCRIPTION OF CRANIAL NERVES

Although several significant approximations to the discovery of nerves were made before the third century BCE, Herophilus must be credited with the first description of the cranial nerves.[3] He first separated the nerves form the arteries and veins and observed that they originated in the brain, the seat of thought. He also demonstrated a differentiation between the nerves capable of sensation and of motion. Even more, he realized that the motor nerves were associated with muscles and that the sensory nerves were associated with the organs of sensation.[4]

In the second century, Galen went a step further in giving the first classification of these cranial nerves.[5] He listed 7 pairs of them, although he actually described 9, a classification that lasted until the seventeenth century.[6,7] To simplify and correlate with modern terminology (not known in that time), Galen did not recognize the olfactory nerve, but did, however, correctly identify the olfactory bulb and tract, which he considered to be an extension of the anterior ventricle. The third pair quite certainly included at least the maxillary and mandibular division of the trigeminal. Concerning the fifth pair, in one text,[8] it consisted in one nerve that divided into 2 parts as it passes through the petrous bone: the hard part, that is, the facial nerve, and the soft part or auditory nerve, that is, the cochleovestibular nerve. In another text,[9] the fifth part was composed of 2 nerves whose individual origins were quite close to one another. The sixth pair was composed of 3 separate nerves, the vagus nerve being better described as the glossopharyngeal. The seventh pair, and last pair of cranial nerves, by Galen designation, is the hypoglossal nerve. Some historians credit Protospatharius[10] for the description of the olfactory nerve in the eighth century.[11] Since the Renaissance, this classification was affined to finally arrive to Soemmerring, in 1778, who introduced the modern 12 pairs for the cranial nerves terminology. If the nerves for olfaction, audition, face, and tongue movements, as well as facial pain were clearly identified, this was not the case for the nerves responsible for gustation. It is only in 1818 that Bellingeri[12] demonstrated that the chorda tympani, a ramus of the VII nerve, was the mediator of taste in the anterior part of the tongue. Much later in the twentieth century, scientists demonstrated that projections of the nerves IX and X also played a role in gustation.

INTRODUCTION OF THE FUNCTIONAL CONCEPT OF ANIMAL SPIRIT

Working at the same time as Herophilus in Alexandria, Erasistratus[13–15] certainly presented the concept of "animal spirit" to explain the function of a nerve. He was the first to postulate a mechanism of brain function.[16] His physiologic system was based on the observation that every organ was equipped with a 3-fold system of vessels or tubes (veins, arteries, and nerves), which are in turn made up of even smaller tubes. Air taken into the lungs went via the heart where it was changed to vital spirits and hence was passed to all parts of the body via the arteries. When the vital spirits reached the brain, they were changed in the cerebral ventricles to animal spirits, originally named "psychic pneuma." The animal spirits were carried to all parts of the body via the hollow nerves.[17]

Galen completely agreed with this explanation and propagated it. He described that the animal spirit, the cerebral spirit, the spirit born in the brain, is the most noble and exquisite part of the human body. This noble spirit is the proper substance of the soul or is, at least, its first instrument.[18] Reason, which in man has its seat in the brain,[19] leads to the ingenious fiction of the birth of the Minerva from the brain of Jupiter.[20] It means that all the productions of the human soul, all arts, and all sciences are born in the brain.[21,22] He thus regarded this animal spirit as deriving its origin from the vital spirit, formed by, or generated in, the heart and arteries. Further he assigned, as the particular source of this secretion, a curious vascular apparatus, known as the *rete mirabile* (retiform plexus).[23,24] This concept was accepted nearly until the eighteenth century. In 1714, Vieussens wrote that "no sensation can occur without the animal spirit being the next and immediate cause."[25]

FIRST ATTEMPTS TO STIMULATE THIS OTOLARYNGOLOGY CRANIAL NERVE ANIMAL SPIRIT, THAT IS, FUNCTIONAL STIMULATION

According to Galen, one of the first attempts to functionally stimulate an OCN was by direct stimulation of the ear sensory peripheral organ with the use of loud sounds by Archigenes in the first century.[26] Even hearing exercises were attempted, but they were fruitless experiments. However, they were to reappear as an acoustic method[27] at the beginning of the twentieth century, when they were hailed as a new miracle method until they vanished again after great disillusionment. In case of facial paralysis, no specific treatment was known since antiquity, except vigorous massages described by Rhazes in the tenth century.[28] It is only at the beginning of the nineteenth century that the facial nerve was recognizable as responsible for facial palsy.[29,30] Nearly until the second part of the eighteenth century, anosmia and agueusia were simply considered as incurable, and no real stimulating treatment was proposed. In 1785, and with taste troubles, "a cure is a desideratum."[31]

In 1790, Vicq-d'Azur proposed to use "sweet and aromatic odor in cases of inertia, to remind the olfactory nerves to their functions."[32] In 1803, "when the sensibility of the nerves which supply the organs of taste is diminished, the chewing of the root of pellitory, horse-radish, or other stimulating substances, will help to recover it."[33] In 1821, Cloquet remarked that abuse of odors might blunt, chafe, and deteriorate olfaction.[34] Functional stimulation of smell and taste seems to have existed at the turn of the nineteenth century, but the literature on these subjects is nearly not existent. In 1890, Rhodes referred to Bosworth who suggested "the employment of agreeable odors, as powerful as can be obtained, changing them frequently, thus stimulating the enfeebled nerves into functional activity."[35]

INTRODUCTION OF ELECTRICAL NERVE IMPULSE THEORY

Since the seventeenth century, the concept of animal spirit began to be questioned and even replaced by other ideas. In 1667, Willis[36] explained that "the animal spirits [...] are irritated into continual, as it were craklings, or convulsive explosions."[37] At the beginning of the eighteenth century, the presence of a "nervous fluid [*fluidum nervosum*]" or "nervous spiritus" is discussed: "There were two opinions on the action of nerves; the one attributes a fluid to these small duct, which arise from the head to the extremities of the nerves; the other give them [...] the same use as the strings of instruments."[38] Another opinion was that "a vibrating electrical virtue can be conveyed and freely act with considerable energy along the surface of animal fibres, and therefore on the nerves."[39] This concept was supported by many physiologists.[40] Nevertheless, in the mid eighteenth century,[41] the ambiguous notions of irritability and sensibility were augmented, notably by Haller.[42] In 1783, Monro explained that "most authors have supposed that the nerves are tubes or ducts conveying a fluid secreted in the brain, cerebellum, and spinal marrow. But, of late years, several ingenious physiologists have contended, that a secreted fluid was too inert for serving the offices performed by the nerves, and, therefore, supposed that they conducted a fluid the same as, or similar to, the electrical fluid."[43]

The existence of an animal spirit was only firmly rejected when scientists began to consider more seriously the nature of electricity.[44(p. 111)] *Electricity* comes from the Green word electron, signifying translucent fossil resin amber. In 1791, Galvani[45] first demonstrated a nonmaterial force with vital properties resembling a form of electricity intrinsic to all living organisms, which he named the "animal electricity [*electricitatis animalis*]".[46] This term was already used in French (*électricité animale*) by Bertholon in 1780.[47(p. 69)] It lead to a fruitful dispute with Volta (artifact of electricity generated by the contact of metal with organic tissue) until 1840 when Matteucci,[48] with the recently invented galvanometer by Schweigger,[49] was able to confirm that an "electrical fluid produces contractions and sensations," in other words, that nerves did indeed contain some type of true biological intrinsic electricity. In the meantime, Cloquet explained that "the nerves that are distributed in the various sense organs are all of the same nature. […] They would make the same feelings if they were also untied, and placed so as to be shaken by the presence of such or such external agent."[50] At the turn of the 1840s, Müller explained that "the laws of action of the nervous principle are totally different from those of electricity."[51] He proposed a theory of specific nerve energies, which stated that different nerves carried a kind of code, which identified their origin to the brain, such as that the sensation of sound must be due to the peculiar energy or quality of the auditory nerve. A step further was added in the 1840s, by Du Bois-Reymond,[52] who discovered in applying an electric shock to an exposed sciatic nerve stump that this produced a decrease in electrical potential that traveled along the surface of the nerve fiber as a wave of relative negativity[44(p. 268)]: "The current-testing device indicates a current that moves from one point to the other, in the direction as they are called […] The nerve current probably touched up one of the primitive nerve tubes […] but the content of it, which appears as a negative element on the cross-section, remains unaffected."[53] This phenomenon of negative variation, which was later named by Hermann "action current,"[54] can be considered as the nerve impulse. Its recognition as an electrical event was revolutionary and opened a new era in the comprehension of nerve function.[55] Helmholtz finally measured the speed of this impulse in 1852[56] at about 30 m/s in stimulating a sciatic frog nerve attached to its muscle.[57] In 1868, Bernstein[58] designed a new instrument, a differential rheotome or current slider, allowing him to more precisely measure the time course of electrical activity in nerve, which was 28.7 m/s.[59] At the beginning of the twentieth century, this electrical activity was called the action potential.

FIRST ELECTRICAL OTOLARYNGOLOGY CRANIAL NERVE STIMULATION DEVICES

The description of the action potential in the nineteenth century led to the development of a new concept of direct nerve stimulation by electricity. Nevertheless, electricity was used already in the second part of the eighteenth century to indistinctly treat various diseases without understanding its mode of action: "Electricity, different from other physical applications, requires rather a nicety of operation than a thorough knowledge of the disease."[60] Although the use of electricity in ancient medicine, from electric catfish, had been depicted many centuries before in ancient Egyptian wall paintings.[61] Hearing was a particular subject to treat with electricity[62] but also "its efficacy in removing the deeper seated pains,"[63] and in nerve palsy. For anosmia, electricity was considered efficient as "a good incisive and an excellent tonic."[47(p. 299)] In 1836, Kramer explained that "I begin with the least curative of all – with a remedy which, from the analogy it has always been believed to possess the power that maintains the nervous influence, was naturally thought also to possess a mightly power of exciting and regulating the nervous influence. In theory, this opinion had everything in its favour; but in practice, even in nervous diseases, the results, in almost all cases in which it was tried, concurred in as loudly condemning it. This is most unequivocally shown in diseases of the ear."[64(p. 53-54)] Kramer also mentioned mineral magnetism[64(p. 65)] and electromagnetism.[65,66] In 1836, Dacamina treated with some success a tongue palsy with galvano-puncture.[67] In 1840, MacKenzie mentioned electricity or galvanism and electropuncture to treat facial palsy.[68]

With the first steps in the understanding of the nerve mode of action in the first part of the nineteenth century, it was evident that a remarkable analogy exists between electricity and the nervous influence: "Electricity acts in a manner peculiar to itself on all the nerves of sensation […] When an electrical current is suddenly transmitted through a nerve to a muscle, or in the inverse direction, the muscle is thrown into spasmodic action."[69] Different forms of electricity[70(p. 12-29)] were then proposed (static electrical current, galvanism,[71,72] voltaism, faradism, d'arsonvalisation, etc.), leading to the production of various man-made electrical devices[73] (**Fig. 1**) with some otolaryngologic indications related to OCN, such as hearing loss, aphonia,[74] "paralysis of portio dura of the seventh pair" that is, facial nerve, neuralgia of the face and of the tongue, stammering, loss of smell and loss of taste,[75] or even anesthesia of trigeminal nerve.[76] Many other otological[77] and pharyngo-laryngological[78] (**Fig. 2**) diseases were also treated leading to a certain overuse of electricity in otolaryngologic therapy.[79–81]

At the beginning of the twentieth century electrotherapy fell from grace, because it lacked a scientific basis and was used also by quacks and charlatans.[82] Nevertheless, new devices were produced such as the Electreat patented in 1919 (**Fig. 3**), as a transcutaneous electrical nerve stimulator to relieve pain.[83,84] The modern electrical

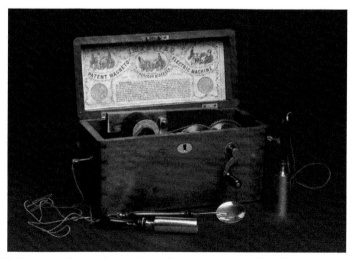

Fig. 1. 1862 Magneto-electrical stimulator. (Image courtesy of Cochlear Americas, ©2019.)

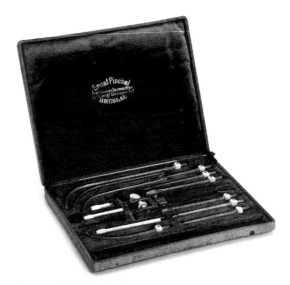

Fig. 2. Galvano-cautery, notably for the larynx.

external stimulators date from the 1940s,[85] but, except for hearing, it took many years before they were used for OCN stimulation.

Olfactory Nerve (Cranial Nerve I)

Anosmia

Early in the nineteenth century there was a dispute of whether smell was facilitated by CN I or CN V. Charles Bell, in 1809, proposed that olfaction was provided by CN I,[86]

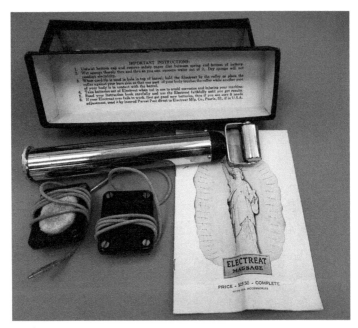

Fig. 3. 1930's Electreat.

with a partially false assumption that CN I and CN V fibers join together for a segment of the projection.[87] However, in 1824, Francois Magendie, through his many series of faulty experiments, suggested that CN V contributed to olfaction,[88] with several studies following right after proving that Bell's theory was indeed partially correct.

The initial studies examining the potential of electrical stimulation (ES) of the olfactory system was done by Schonbein in 1851, who suggested that people can smell the electric discharge.[89] Aronsohn also reported on perceiving odor through electricity.[90] Almost a century later, in 1961, Yamamoto studied the ES of the olfactory mucosa in a rabbit.[91] ES of olfactory mucosa, in case of postoperative anosmia (after removal of olfactory nerve), was tried in 1970,[92] and in 1983 it was concluded that stimulation of human olfactory nerves did not evoke the sensation of smell, but suppressed smell sensations of presented odorants.[93,94] Later experiment in 2012 demonstrated that definitely ES can stimulate the smell sensations. Kumar and colleagues showed that ES of the olfactory bulb and tract produced various smells, both pleasant and unpleasant, in epilepsy patients.[95] With further modifications in the application of electrical current in 2018, induction of smell through transethmoid ES was possible.[96]

Trigeminal Nerve (Cranial Nerve V)

Facial pain
Bausch in 1672 and later Fothergill in 1773 described tic douloureux as an extremely disabling illness[97] that sometimes has been termed a suicide disease.[98] The most common causes of facial pain include trigeminal neuralgia and trigeminal neuropathic pain, both of which are characterized by severe facial neuropathic pain in one or more of the trigeminal nerve divisions, with latter having an additional symptom of constant burning pain. Wall and Sweet in 1967 described using ES of peripheral trigeminal nerve as a treatment of neuropathic pain.[99] Shelden (1966) also reported on relief of trigeminal neuralgia by ES of the trigeminal ganglion.[100] Although results of ES of trigeminal ganglion were favorable, many reports were of short duration with inadequate stimulation coverage of the nerve. Cook and team experimented with more permanent methods of ES for facial neuralgia.[101] Besides ES, facial pain treatment included microvascular decompression, developed by Jannetta.[102] Even deep brain stimulation was tried for intractable pain.[103]

Facial Nerve (Cranial Nerve VII)

Facial nerve paralysis
In 1841, Reid suggested that ES of denervated muscle could offset the structural and physiologic changes that ensue from loss of motor innervation.[104] Use of galvanism during these years was part of daily medical practice and electric current application to paralyzed limbs was common.[70(p. 72)] Botelho and colleagues[105] in 1952 first reported on ES of the facial nerve at the stylomastoid foramen to elicit a compound muscle action potential. Not long has passed that patient's with facial nerve palsy, Bell palsy, began to receive ES of the facial nerve with hopes of improving recovery and preserving muscle tone.

A controlled trial was done by Mosforth and Tavern (1958) to use ES of facial nerve as a treatment of Bell palsy. In their study, ES, in addition to daily facial massage as compared with massage alone, was concluded to neither cause harm nor benefit in patients affected by Bell palsy.[106] Later both Farragher and colleagues[107] (1987) and Targan and colleagues[108] (2000) tried modification of ES by applying either "eutrophic" stimulation or using pulsed ES, respectively, and although some improvement in motor dysfunction was observed in patients with Bell palsy, both studies lacked control groups, making it hard to assess causality of treatment. Later studies also examined other therapies for facial nerve recovery, including EMG-biofeedback compared with mirror-feedback and[109] small-movement therapy as compared with facial exercise.[110] Moreover, recently some improvement in facial outcomes have been reported with the use of mime therapy.[111]

Cochleovestibular Nerve (Cranial Nerve VIII)

Audition

Attempts at ES of the auditory apparatus began with Veratti[112,113] and Wilson[114] who applied extrauricular ES since 1747, to deafened persons. However, following Wilson's experiments on an additional 6 individuals yielded no further benefit. Not long after Volta in 1790, through self-experimentation, connected a battery of 50V (**Fig. 4**) to 2 metal rods and inserted it into his ears, it stimulated cranial nerves. He reported experiencing auditory stimulation by "hearing a *sound, or rather noise in the ears, which I cannot well define…*" describing it as a blow to the head followed by a sound of boiling of a viscid liquid.[115] Intermittent reports followed over the next half of the century with the assumption that the acoustic perception resulted directly from stimulation of the acoustic nerve.[116] The latter half of the century differed, as it embraced the concept that it was more the stimulation of current on the ossicles and the tympanic membrane, the conductive apparatus, that led to perceived sound awareness. Nevertheless, by 1868 Brunner demonstrated in his systematic study the use of ES of the auditory system.[77(p. 230)] With this a new field of treatment of ear

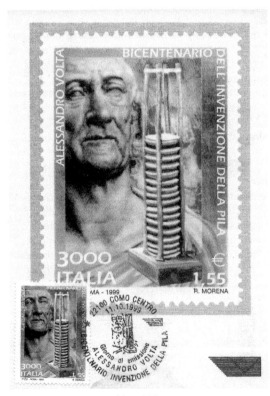

Fig. 4. Volta battery. Italian stamp issued in 1999.

pathologies arose, termed "electro-otiatrics," with common ear pathologies such as otitis media and tinnitus receiving ES as part of a treatment of the disease.[117] These early experimentations, however, were relatively naïve in a comparator to studies developed in the late twentieth century. In 1957, Djourno and Eyries performed the first experiment by directly applying ES to the auditory nerve in a deaf person.[118] From this research the creation of first CI and auditory brainstem implant, as a surgical intervention for the deaf, emerged.

Vestibular

Gernandt and collegues[119] in 1957 described ES of the whole vestibular nerve. Cohen and his team reported, in their work of stimulation by a single as well as multielectrode of vestibular nerve branches, its effect on direction of nystagmus.[120] The success of the CI in treating hearing loss has led to the development of vestibular implant. Gong and Merfeld first described a single-channel prototype of this device.[121] Since then, several outcomes of vestibular implant have been described in literature.

Glossopharyngeal Nerve (Cranial Nerve IX)

Paralysis of the palate

Although a relatively understudied area, palatal ES to cure palatal paralysis has been described. Palate receives innervation from branches of both glossopharyngeal and vagus nerves. Gessler (1889) and Sajous (1894)[122,123] reported on a use of ES and cure for palatal paralysis. Use of galvanic current application can be later seen for the treatment of palatal paralysis in a lateral medullary syndrome with success.[124] Although some showed that palatal ES did not affect swallowing[125] measures, others demonstrated that indeed they had significant improvement in function in patients with acute stroke.[126,127]

Vagal Nerve (Cranial Nerve X)

Vocal cord paralysis

Sushruta first mentioned anatomic structures contributing to voice in the sixth century BC in India. He described 4 arteries, 2 on each side of the windpipe, with one pair being that of glistening white structure, whereas the other pair being purple. Sushruta reported that injury to either one around the area of the trachea produced dumbness and change in voice.[128] Thus, initially it was injury to vessels that was considered to cause hoarseness. However, it was during the second century AD, where Galen, in a pig model, demonstrated and described in detail the course of the recurrent laryngeal nerve, a branch of vagal nerve that innervates the larynx.[129] In his research, he showed that pigs that had their nerve severed were unable to squeal. Galen also described the same effect in one infant who had undergone surgery for goiter and had aphonia (ie, vocal cord paralysis).[130,131] The first 2 to apply ES in the form of galvanic and faradic current to the musculature of the larynx, by applying ES to the thyroid cartilage, were Rossbach (1881)[132] and Gerhardt (1884).[133,134] In its initial stage transcutaneous stimulation of laryngeal nerve was thought to be difficult by von Ziemssen[135] whereas King believed it was possible.[136] Direct stimulation of recurrent laryngeal nerve was reported in the first part of the twentieth century.[137,138] The first experiment of transcutaneous ES of the nerve did not happen until 1986 by Sanders, who published an experiment in dogs with transcutaneous ES initiating vocal cord movement,[139] and more recently investigations of transcutaneous ES of branches of vagal nerve have been evaluated.[140]

Seizures and tinnitus

Although Parry was the first to use carotid massage for treatment of nervous disorders,[141,142] it was Corning who first applied ES to stimulate the vagal nerve.[143] His initial experiments of manually compressing the carotid arteries during seizure made him realize the need to stimulate CN X as an abortive treatment of seizures. However, the frustration of having to hold the neck with the patient and musculature of the cervical neck contracting violently, during a seizure, modified his technique to transcutaneous electrical vagal nerve stimulation and a carotid compression device. ES studies on vagal nerve were conducted during the 1930s and 1940s and demonstrated that stimulation of vagal nerve influenced brain electrical activity and had anticonvulsant effects. After many trials in 1997, a vagal nerve stimulator device was approved for the treatment of refractory epilepsy.[144] More recently vagal nerve stimulator has been used for the treatment of tinnitus when paired with brief pulsed ES of the vagus nerve.[145]

Taste

Taste is transmitted to the brain through 3 cranial nerves: CN VII from the anterior two-thirds of the tongue, CN IX from posterior one-third part of the tongue, and CN X nerve from the back of the oral cavity. In 1754, Sulzer described a way of inducing taste as that of ferrous sulphate was induced by 2 different, interconnected metals touched by the tongue.[146] Later, Allen and Weinberg (1925) reported on vibrating taste sensations.[147] Electrophysiologic experiments of chorda tympani (a branch of facial nerve) fibers demonstrated that taste (sweet, salty, sour, and bitter) is encoded neutrally. Direct stimulation of chorda tympani was done in the early twentieth century,[148–150] and over the later part, various ways of stimulating taste were tried, including salt stimulation,[151] pulsatile stimulation,[152] thermal stimulation,[153] and stimulation with solutions of metal salts and with metal and electrical currents.[154] Electrogustometer was developed to stimulate gustatory receptors to measure taste thresholds using ES directly on the tongue.[155,156] This was followed by transcranial magnetic stimulation[157] and stimulation with cold.[158] Nevertheless, no clinically relevant ES implantable stimulator for taste restoration is currently used in clinical practice.

Hypoglossal Nerve (Cranial Nerve XII)

Sleep apnea

Research in stimulation of the tongue proper and hypoglossal nerve for the treatment of upper airway obstruction is relatively new, although tongue was stimulated before for experiments on awake dogs by stimulating genioglossus with direct needle electrode insertion, with first publication from a group in Japan in 1988.[159] In humans, similar attempts were made by Guilleminault through transcutaneous submental and intraoral ES, although the results were unsuccessful.[160] Thus Miki and colleagues[161,162] performed transcutaneous submental stimulation while looking at polysomnographic studies with evidence of reducing obstructive sleep apnea symptoms. Later Eisele and Schwartz (1993) tested the application of ES to the hypoglossal nerve for treatment of upper airway obstruction.[163,164] This research gave rise to advancement and application of ES in implantable hypoglossal nerve stimulator (HNS) that is now used to treat intractable sleep apnea.

DEVELOPMENT OF CRANIAL NERVE–IMPLANTED STIMULATORS IN OTOLARYNGOLOGY

In the mid-twentieth century, a new concept of ES was developed, the idea being to replace the peripheral sensory receptor, in other words, to enable the brain to interpret this modified ES as a sensory input. Although many experiments of ES on OCN have been performed, as described earlier, a small minority went on to have a development of an implantable device that would stimulate the nerve on a constant basis with clinically significant implications. In fact, to date, patients derive benefits from a CI to restore hearing and in rare cases to suppress perverse tinnitus,[165] a hypoglossal nerve stimulator to treat intractable sleep apnea, and although a vagal nerve stimulator device was approved for the treatment of refractory epilepsy, its use within the field of otolaryngology as an implantable device is still limited.

William F. House is credited for implanting the first CI in 1961.[166–168] It was not long after that the first child received a CI in 1980.[169] CI was originally developed for adults and children with profound sensorineural hearing loss, but indications, since its initial Food and Drug Administration approval in 1984, have expanded to include a broader patient population[170] (**Fig. 5**). However, although CI is able to improve hearing for many, there is still a subset of deaf patients that would derive little to no benefit from a CI. This led to the advent of auditory brainstem implant, which was designed to stimulate the cochlear nucleus in the brainstem for those individuals lacking a viable auditory nerve. Implantation of the first auditory brainstem implant was performed in 1979 by House and Hitselberger in an adult with neurofibromatosis type 2 (NF2)[171] and received its Food and Drug Administration (FDA) approval in the year 2000 for patients with NF2 12 years and older. With changes in the implant candidacy more adult and children now qualify to receive an implant. Although many are able to derive great benefit in postimplant hearing outcomes, there are still those that do not derive benefit. Within the research field, focusing on identifying preimplant predictors can recognize CI candidates who may be at high risk for a poor outcome following implantation.

HNS is a relatively new device, with increased attention in recent years. It is currently used as a treatment option for CPAP refractory obstructive sleep apnea. The first HNS device was developed by Medtronic in the early 1990s. It was initially a radio

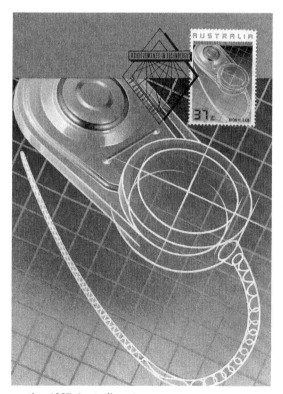

Fig. 5. CI commemorative 1987 Australian stamp.

frequency controlled device with external apparatus that provided ES to the hypoglossal nerve. With further modifications, the first fully implantable close-loop system was developed subsequently by Inspire Medical Systems and is often referred to as inspire device. Initial clinical trial results were published in 2001[172] and gained approval by the FDA in 2014. The approval of the device was based on a pivotal trial, Stimulation Therapy for Apnea Reduction (STAR),[173] examining 126 patients with obstructive sleep apnea after HNS implantation. The STAR trial patients have been closely observed, and recent 5-year follow-up demonstrates sustainable results.[174]

SUMMARY

The history that led to the development of currently used implantable OCN stimulators in Otolaryngology is rich and extends over centuries. Although ES has been applied to many OCN, only few implantable devices were developed with current clinical use. There is still a large window of opportunity and need to develop novel devices in the future.

DISCLOSURE

None.

REFERENCES

1. Soemmerring ST. De basi encephali et originibus nervorum cranio egredentium libri quinque. Goettingae: Vandenhoeck; 1778.
2. Corrales CE, Mudry A, Jackler RK. Perpetuation of errors in illustrations of cranial nerve anatomy. J Neurosurg 2017;127(1):192–8.
3. Von Staden H. Herophilus the art of medicine in early Alexandria. Cambridge (England): University Press; 1998. p. 159.
4. Panegyres KP, Panegyres PK. The ancient Greek discovery of the nervous system: alcmaeon, praxagoras and herophilus. J Clin Neurosci 2016;29:21–4.
5. Spillane JD. The doctrine of the nerves. Oxford (England): University Press; 1981. p. 19–20.
6. Smith ES. Galen's account of the cranial nerves and the autonomic nervous system. 1. Clio Med 1971;6(2):77–98.
7. Smith ES. Galen's account of the cranial nerves and the autonomic nervous system. 2. Clio Med 1971;6(3):173–94.
8. Galenus C. De usu partium corporis humani, IX, 10. In: Kühn CG, editor. Galeni Opera omnia, vol. III. Leipzig (Germany): Cnoblochii; 1822. p. 723.
9. Galenus C. De nervorum dissectione, VI. In: Kühn CG, editor. Galeni Opera omnia, vol. II. Leipzig (Germany): Cnoblochii; 1821. p. 837–8.
10. Protospatharius T. De corporis humani fabrica libri V. Venetiis; 1536. p. 71.
11. Willemot J. Naissance et développement de l'oto-rhino-laryngologie dans l'histoire de la médecine. Acta Otorhinolaryngol Belg 1981;(Suppl):1–1698, 1062.
12. Bellingeri CF. Dissertatio inauguralis… Quinti, et septimi paris functiones. Augustae Taurinorum (Italy): Favale; 1818. p. 170.
13. Christie RV. Galen on Erasistratus. Perspect Biol Med 1987;30(3):440–9.
14. Pearce JMS. The neurology of Erasistratus. J Neurol Disord 2013;1:1–3.
15. Smith CUM, Frixione E, Finger S, et al. The animal spirit doctrine and the origins of neurophysiology. Oxford (England): University Press; 2012. p. 33.
16. Longrigg J. Greek rational medicine. London: Routledge; 1993. p. 211–5.

17. McHenry LC. Garrison's history of neurology. Springfield (MA): Thomas; 1969. p. 12.
18. Galenus C. De usu respirationis, 5. In: Kühn CG, editor. Galeni Opera omnia, vol. IV. Leipzig (Germany): Cnoblochii; 1822. p. 501–2.
19. Galenus C. De usu partium corporis humani, IV, 13. In: Kühn CG, editor. Galeni Opera omnia, vol. III. Leipzig (Germany): Cnoblochii; 1822. p. 309.
20. Johnston C. A lecture upon the discovery of the circulation of the blood and the theories of generation. Am J Dent Sci 1857;7:157–83.
21. Galenus C. De Hippocratis et Platonis decretis, III, 8. In: Kühn CG, editor. Galeni Opera omnia, vol. V. Leipzig (Germany): Cnoblochii; 1823. p. 348.
22. Flourens P. Histoire de la découverte de la circulation du sang. 2nd edition. Paris: Garnier; 1857. p. 92.
23. Galenus C. De usu partium corporis humani, IX, 4. In: Kühn CG, editor. Galeni Opera omniavol. III. Leipzig (Germany): Cnoblochii; 1822. p. 696.
24. Pettigrew TJ. Biographical memoirs of the most celebrated physicians, surgeons, etc. London: Whittaker & Co; 1839. p. 8. Galen.
25. Vieussens R. Traité nouveau de la structure de l'oreille. Toulouse (France): Guillemette; 1714. p. 90.
26. Galenus C. De compositione medicamentorum secundum locos III, 1. In: Kühn CG, editor. Galeni Opera omnia, vol. XII. Leipzig (Germany): Cnoblochii; 1826. p. 655–6.
27. Goldstein M. The acoustic method for the training of the deaf and hard-of-hearing child. St Louis (MO): Laryngoscope; 1939.
28. Pearce JMS. Early observations on facial palsy. J Hist Neurosci 2015;24:319–25.
29. Bell C. On the nerves; giving an account of some experiments on their structure and functions, which lead t a new arrangement of the system. Phil Trans Roy Soc Lond 1821;111:398–424.
30. Glicenstein J. Histoire de la paralysie faciale. Ann Chir Plast Esthet 2015;60: 347–62.
31. Motherby G. A new medical dictionary. 2nd edition. London: Johnson; 1785. gustus.
32. Vicq-d'Azur F. Encyclopédie méthodique, vol. III. Paris: Panckoucke; 1790. p. 47.
33. Anonymous. New edition. The Edinburgh practice of physic, surgery, and midwifery, vol. II. London: Kearsley; 1803. p. 527.
34. Cloquet H. Osphrésiologie, ou traité des odeurs, du sens et des organes de l'olfaction. 2nd ediiton. Paris: Méquignon-Marvis; 1821. p. 751.
35. Rhodes JE. Anosmia. Chicago: Medical Press; 1890. p. 7.
36. Willis T. Pathologiae cerebri et nervosi generis specimen. Hall (FL): Oxonii; 1667. p. 114.
37. Schechter DS. Origins of electrotherapy. Part II. N Y State J Med 1971;71(10): 1114–24.
38. Anonymous. Physical essays on the parts of the human body. London: Clarke; 1734. p. 396.
39. Hales S. Statical essays: containing haemastaticks, vol. II. London: Innys & Co; 1733. p. 59.
40. Verkhratsky A, Parpura V. History of electrophysiology and the patch clamp. In: Msrtins M, Taverna S, editors. Patch-clamp methods and protocols. 2nd edition. New York: Springer; 2014. p. 1–19.
41. Boury D. Irritability and sensibility: key concepts in assessing the medical doctrines of Haller and Bordeu. Sci Context 2008;21(4):521–35.
42. Haller A. Dissertation sur les parties irritables et sensibles des animaux. Lausanne (Switzerland): Bousquet; 1755.

43. Monro A. Observations on the structures and functions of the nervous system. Edinburgh (Scotland): Creech; 1783. p. 74.
44. Wickens AP. A history of the brain. London: Psychology Press; 2015. p. 111, 268.
45. Piccolino M. Animal electricity and the birth of electrophysiology: the legacy of Luigi Galvani. Brain Res Bull 1998;5:381–407.
46. Galvani L. De viribus electricitatis in motu musculari commentarius. Bononiae (Italy): Instituti Scientiarum; 1791. p. 17.
47. Bertholon A. De l'électricité du corps humain dans l'état de santé et de maladie. Lyon (France): Bernuset; 1780. p. 69, 299.
48. Matteucci C. Essai sur les phénomènes électriques des animaux. Paris: Carillan-Goeury & Dalmont; 1840. p. 37.
49. Schweigger JSC. Noch einige Worte über diese neuen elektromagnetischen Phänomene. J Chem Phys 1821;31:35–41.
50. Cloquet H. Système anatomique, vol. II. Paris: Agasse; 1825. p. 518.
51. Müller J. Elements of physiology, vol. I. London: Taylor & Walton; 1842. p. 640.
52. Meltzer SJ. Emil du Bois-Reymond. Science 1897;5(110):217–9.
53. Du Bois-Reymond E. Vorläufiger Abris seiner Untersuchung über den sogenannten Froschstrom und über die elektromotorische Fische. Poggendorff's Ann Phys Chem 1843;58:1–30.
54. Hermann L. Untersuchungen zur Physiologie der Muskeln und Nerven, vol. III. Berlin: Hirschwald; 1868. p. 61.
55. Finkelstein G. Mechnanical neuroscience: Emil du Bois-Reymond's innovations in theory and practice. Front Syst Neurosci 2015;9:133.
56. Helmholtz H. Messungen über Fortpflanzungsgeschwindigkeit der Reizung in den Nerven. Arch Anat Physiol Wiss Med 1852;199–216.
57. Glickstein M. Neuroscience. A historical introduction. Cambridge (England): MIT Press; 2014. p. 59.
58. Berstein J. Ueber den zeitlichen Verlauf der negative Schwankung des Nervenstroms. Pflugers Arch 1868;1:173–207.
59. Seyfarth EA. Julius Bernstein (1839-1917) : pioneer neurobiologist and biophysicist. Biol Cybern 2006;94:2–8.
60. Cavallo T. An essay on the theory and practice of medical electricity. London: Author; 1781. p. 5.
61. Howes GJ. The phylogenetic relationships of the electric catfish family malapteruridae (Teleostei: Siluroidei). J Nat Hist 1985;19:37–67.
62. Rowbottom M, Susskind C. Electricity and medicine. History of their interaction. San Francisco (CA): San Francisco Press; 1984. p. 15–30.
63. Wilkinson CH. The effects of electricity. London: Allen; 1799. p. 11.
64. Kramer W. Die Erkenntniss und Heilung der Ohrenkrankheiten. Berlin: Nicolai; 1836. p. 53–4, 65.
65. Kramer W. Beiträge zur Ohrenheilkunde. Berlin: Nicolai; 1845. p. 245.
66. O'Connor ME, Bentall RHC, Monahan JC. Emerging electromagnetic medicine. New York: Springer; 1990.
67. Anonymous. Palsy of the tongue cured by galvano-puncture. J Psychol Med 1849;2:162.
68. MacKenzie W. A practical treatise on the diseases of the eye. 3rd edition. London: Longman & Co; 1840. p. 149.
69. Fischer GT. A practical treatise on medical electricity. London: Willats; 1845. p. 21–3.
70. Channing WF. Notes on the medical application of electricity. Boston: Davis; 1849. p. 12–29, 72.

71. Finger S, Piccolino M, Stahnisch FW. Alexander von Humboldt: Galvanism, animal electrictiy, and self-experimentation. Part 1. J Hist Neurosci 2013;22: 225–60.
72. Finger S, Piccolino M, Stahnisch FW. Alexander von Humboldt: Galvanism, animal electrictiy, and self-experimentation. Part 2. J Hist Neurosci 2013;22: 327–52.
73. Meyer M. Die Electricität in ihrer Anwendung auf practische Medizin. Berlin: Hirschwald; 1854. p. 50–67.
74. Aphonia cured by galvanism. Lancet 1843;40(1030):291–2.
75. Althaus J. A treatrise on medical electricity. Philadelphia: Lindsay & Blakiston; 1860. p. 312–4.
76. Erb W. Handbuch der Elektrotherapie. Leipzig (Germany): Vogel; 1882. p. 548.
77. Brenner R. Untersuchungen und Beobachtungen über die Wirkung elektrischer Ströme auf das Gehörorgan. Leipzig (Germany): Giesecke & Devrient; 1868. p. 230.
78. Voltolini R. Die Anwendung der Galvanokaustik im inner des Kehlkopfes und Schlundkopfes. Wien (Austria): Braumüller; 1867.
79. Scheppegrell W. Electricity in the diagnosis and treatment of diseases of the nose, throat and ear. New York: Putnam; 1898.
80. Coleman WF. Electricity in diseases of the eye, ear, nose and throat. Lincoln (IL): Courier-Herald Press; 1912.
81. Lermoyez M. Notions pratiques d'électricité à l'usage des médecins avec renseignements spéciaux pour les oto-rhino-laryngologistes. Paris: Masson; 1913.
82. Heidland A, Fazeli G, Klassen A, et al. Neuromuscular electrostimulation techniques: historical aspects and current possibilities in treatment of pain and muscle waisting. Clin Nephrol 2013;79(Suppl 1):S12–23.
83. Slavin KV. History of peripheral nerve stimulation. Prog Neurol Surg 2011; 24:1–15.
84. Shealy CN. Transcutaneous electrical nerve stimulation: the treatment of choice for pain and depression. J Altern Complement Med 2003;9(5):619–23.
85. Geddes LA. The first stimulators-reviewing the history of electrical stimulation and the devices crucial to its development. IEEE Eng Med Biol 1994;13(4): 532–42.
86. Bell C. The anatomy of the human body, vol. III. New York: Collins & Perkins; 1809. p. 84.
87. Bell C. Idea of a new anatomy of the brain. Facsimile of an article of 1811. London: Dawsons of Pall Mall; 1966. p. 28.
88. Magendie F. Le nerf olfactif estil l'organe de l'odorat ? Expériences sur cette question. J Physiol Exp Pathol 1824;4:169–76.
89. Schönbein CF. On some secondary physiological effects produced by atmospheric electricity. Med Chir Trans 1851;1:205–20.
90. Aronsohn E. Ueber elektrische Geruchtempfindung. Arch Physiol 1884;8:460–5.
91. Yamamoto C. Olfactory bulb potentials to electrical stimulation of the olfactory mucosa. Jpn J Physiol 1961;11(5):545–54.
92. Orlandi F, Alvisi C, Serra D, et al. L'elettrostimulazione della mucosa olfattiva in soggetti con anosmia postoperative. Folia Endocrinol 1970;23(3):307–13.
93. Straschill M, Stahl H, Gorkisch K. Effects of electrical stimulation of the human olfactory mucosa. Appl Neurophysiol 1983;46:286–9.
94. Gorkisch K, Axhausen M, Straschill M. Elektrische Stimulation des menschlichen N. olfactorius – ein Zugant zum Kurzzeitgedächtnis. HNO 1985;33(1):325–7.

95. Kumar G, Juhasz C, Sood S, et al. Olfactory hallucinations elicited by electrical stimulation via subdural eleectrodes: effects of direct stimulation of olfactory bulb and tract. Epilepsy Behav 2012;24(2):264–8.
96. Holbrook EH, Puram SV, See RB, et al. Induction of smell through transethmoid electrical stimulation of the olfactory bulb. Int Forum Allergy Rhinol 2019;9: 158–64.
97. Stookey B, Ransohoff J. Trigeminal neuralgia. Its history and treatment. Springfield (MA): Thomas; 1959.
98. Eboli P, Stones JL, Audin S, et al. Historical characterization of trigeminal neuralgia. Neurosurgery 2009;64:1183–7.
99. Wall PD, Sweet WH. Temporal abolition of pain in man. Science 1967;155(3758): 108–9.
100. Shelden CH. Depolarization in the treatment of trigeminal neuralgia. In: Knighton RS, Dumke PR, editors. Pain. Boston: Little Brown; 1966. p. 373–86.
101. Cook AW, Zandieh M, Baggenstos P, et al. Radiofrequency stimulation of the trigeminal complex in tic douloureux and atypical facial neuralgia: temporary percutaneous and permanent methods. Acupunct Electrother Res 1978;3: 37–47.
102. Jannetta PJ, McLAughlin MR, Casey KF. Technique of microvascular decompression. Neurosurg Focus 2005;18:1–5.
103. Boccard SGJ, Pereira EAC. Deep brain stimulation for chronic pain. J Clin Neurosci 2015;22(10):1537–43.
104. Reid J. On the relation between muscular contractility and the nervous system. Lond Eding Month J Med Sci 1841;1:320–9.
105. Botelho, Deaterly CF, Comroe JH. Electrmyogram from orbicularis oculi in normal persons and patients with myasthenia gravis. AMA Arch Neurol Psychiatry 1952;67:348–53.
106. Mosforth J, Taverned D. Physiotherapy for Bell's palsy. BMJ 1958;2(5097): 675–7.
107. Farragher D, Kidd GL, Tallis R. Eutrophic electrical stimulation for Bell's palsy. Clin Rehabil 1987;1(4):265–71.
108. Targan R, Alon G, Kay SL. Effect of long-term electrical stimulation on motor recovery and improvement of clinical residuals in patients with unresolved facial nerve palsy. Otolaryngol Head Neck Surg 2000;122:246–52.
109. Ross B, Nedzelski JM, Mclean JA. Efficacy of feedback training in long standing facial nerve paresis. Laryngoscope 1991;101:744–50.
110. Segal B, hunter T, Danys I, et al. Minimizing synkinesis during rehabilitation of the paralyzed face: preliminary assessment of a new small-movement therapy. Am J Otolaryngol 1995;24:149–53.
111. Beurskens CHG, Devriese PD, Heiningen I, et al. The use of mine therapy as a rehabilitation method for patients with facial nerve paresis. Inter J Therap Rehab 2004;11(5):206–10.
112. Veratti G. Osservazioni fisico-mediche intorno alla elettricita. Bologna (Italy): della Volpe; 1748.
113. Marchese-Ragona R, Pendolino AL, Mudry A, et al. The father of the electrical stimulation of the ear. Otol Neurotol 2019;40:404–6.
114. Wilson B. A treatrise on electricity. 2nd edition. London: Davis; 1752. p. 202–8.
115. Volta A. On the electricity excited by mere contact of conducting substances of different kinds. Trans Roy Soc Phil 1800;90:403–31.
116. Scheppegrell W. Electricity in diseases of the nose, throat and ear. New York: Putman; 1898. p. 315–25.

117. Neftel WB. Galvano-Therapeutics. New York: Appleton; 1871. p. 9.
118. Djourno A, Eyries C. Prothèse auditive par excitation électrique à distance du nerf sensoriel à l'aide d'un bobinage inclus à demeure. Presse Med 1957; 65(63):1417.
119. Gernandt BE, Katsuki Y, Andlivingston RB. Functional organization of descending vestibular influences. J Neurophysiol 1957;20:453–69.
120. Cohen B, Suzuki J-I, Bender ME. Eye movements from semicircular canal stimulation in the cat. Ann Otol Rhinol Laryngol 1964;73:153–69.
121. Gong W, Merfeld DM. Prototype neural semicircular canal prosthesis using patterned electrical stimulation. Ann Biomed Eng 2000;28(5):572–81.
122. Gessler H. Electrotherapeutische Erfahrungen. Med Correspondenzblatt Wurtemberg Arztliches Landesvereins, 1889;35.
123. Sajous CE. Diseases of the nose, naso-pharynx, pharynx, and larynx. In: Bigelow HR, editor. An international system of electro-therapeutics. Philadelphia: Davis; 1894. I-1 – I-36.
124. Ghatak RK, Choudhury BK, Ballav A, et al. Role of electrical stimulation of palate in patients of lateral medullary syndrome with dysphagia. IJPMR 2006; 17(2):45–8.
125. Power M, Fraser C, Hobson A, et al. Changes in pharyngeal corticobulbar excitatbility and swallowing behavior after oral stimulation. Am J Physiol Gastrointest Liver Physiol 2004;286(1):G45–50.
126. Fraser C, Power M, Hamdy S, et al. Driving plasticity in human adult motor cortex is associated with improved motor function after brain injury. Neuron 2002; 34(5):831–40.
127. Jayasekeran V, Singh S, Tyrell P, et al. Adjunctive functional pharyngeal electrical stimulation reverses swallowing disability after brain lesions. Gastroenterology 2010;138(5):1737–46.
128. Bhishagratna KJ. The Susruta Samhita, vol. I. Varanasi (India): Chowkhamba; 1998. p. 185.
129. Galenus C. On anatomical procedures. In: Lyons MC, Towers B, editors. Cambridge (England): University Press; 1962. p. 81. Transl. by Duckworth WLH.
130. Galenus C. De locis affectis liber I, 6. In: Kühn CG, editor. Galeni Opera omnia, vol. VIII. Leipzig (Germany): Cnoblochii; 1824. p. 48.
131. Wright J. The nose and throat in the history of medicine. Laryngoscope 1901;11: 173–96.
132. Rossbach MJ. Ueber Behandlung und Heilung der Kehlkopf Schwindsucht. In: Verbindung mit E. Sehrwald, editor. Gesammelte Klinische Arbeiten, vol. iv. Jena (Germany): Fischer; 1890. p. 48–53.
133. Gerhardt C. Studien und Beobachtungen über Stimmbandlähmung. Virchow Arch Pathol Anat Physiol 1863;27:68–98.
134. Althaus J. A treatise on medical electricity. 3rd edition. London: Longmans, Green, & Co; 1873. p. 421.
135. Ziemssen H. Die Electricität in der Medicin. 3rd edition. Berlin: Hirschwald; 1866. p. 68.
136. King WH. The development of the higher vocal register by electricity. Homoeopathic Eye Ear Throat J 1896;2(12):392.
137. Nakamura F. Movement of the larynx induced by electrical stimulation of the laryngeal nerve. In: Brewer DW, editor. Research potentials in voice physiology. Syracuse (NY): New York State University Press; 1961. p. 129–36.
138. Erlanger J, Gasser HS. The action potential in fibers of slow conduction in spinal root and somatic nerves. Am J Physiol 1930;92:43–82.

139. Sanders I, Aviv J, biller HF. Transcutaneous electrical stimulation of the recurrent laryngeal nerve: a method of controlling vocal cord position. Otolaryngol Head Neck Surg 1986;95(2):152–7.

140. Seifpanahi S, Izadi F, Jamshidi AA, et al. Effects of transcutaneous electrical stimulation on vocal folds adduction. Eur Arch Otorhinolaryngol 2017;274(9):3423–8.

141. Parry CH. On the effects of compression of the arteries in various diseases, and particularly in those of the head; with hints towards a new mode of treating nervous disorders. Mem Med Soc Lond 1792;3:77–113.

142. Parry CH. On a case of nervous affection cured by pressure of the carotids: with some physiological remarks. Phil Trans Roy Soc Lond 1811;1:89–95.

143. Corning JL. Electrization of the sympathetic and pneumogastric nerves, with simultaneous bilateral compression of the carotids. New York Med J 1884;39:212–5.

144. Morris GL, Gloss D, Buchhalter J, et al. Evidence-based guideline update: vagus nerve stimulation of the treatment of epilepsy. Neurology 2013;81:1453–9.

145. Tyler R, Cacace A, Stocking C, et al. Vagus nerve stimulation paired with tones for the treatment of tinnitus: A prospective randomized double-blind controlled pilot study in humans. Sci Rep 2017;7(1):11960.

146. Bujas Z. Electrical taste. In: Beidler L, editor. Handbook of sensory physiology, vol. IV, 2. Berlin: Springer; 1971. p. 180–99.

147. Allen F, Weinberg M. The gustatory sensory reflex. Q J Exp Physiol 1923;15:385–420.

148. Pfaffmann C. Gustatory afferent impulses. J Cell Comp Physiol 1941;17:242–58.

149. Eliasson S, Gisselsson L. Electrical stimulation of chorda tympani in human being. Acta Otolaryngol Suppl 1954;116:72–5.

150. Frenckner P, Preber L. The effect of electrical stimulation of the chorda tympani. Acta Otolaryngol Suppl 1954;116:100–4.

151. Beidler LM. A theory of taste stimulation. J Gen Physiol 1954;38(2):133–9.

152. Meiselman HL, Halpern BP. Enhancement of taste intensity through pulsatile stimulation. Physiol Behav 1973;11:713–6.

153. Cruz A, Green BG. Thermal stimulation of taste. Nature 2000;403:889–92.

154. Lawless HT, Stevens DA, Chapman KW, et al. Metallic taste from electrical and chemical stimulations. Chem Senses 2005;30(3):185–94.

155. Frank ME, Hettinger TF, Herness MS, et al. Evaluation of taste function by electrogustometry. In: Meisselman HR, Rivlin RS, editors. Clinical measurement of taste and smell. New York: MacMillan; 1986. p. 187–99.

156. McClure ST, Lawless HT. A comparison of two electrical taste stimulation devices. Physiol Behav 2007;92(4):658–64.

157. Henkin RI, Potolicchio SJ, Levy LM. Improvement in smell and taste dysfunction after repetitive transcranial magnetic stimulation. Am J Otolaryngol 2010;32:38–46.

158. Fujiyama R, Toda K. Functional effects of cold stimulation on taste perception in humans. Odontology 2017;105(3):275–82.

159. Miki H, Hida W, Shindoh C, et al. Effects of electrical stimulation of the genioglossus on upper airway resistance in anesthetized dogs. Am Rev Respir Dis 1989;140:1279–84.

160. Guilleminault C, Hill MW, Simmons FB, et al. Obstructive sleep apnea: electromyographic and fiberoptic studies. Exp Neurol 1978;62:48–67.

161. Miki H, Hida W, Inmoue H, et al. A new treatment for obstructive sleep apnea syndrome by electrical stimulation of submental region. Tohoku J Exp Med 1988;154:91–2.
162. Miki H, Hida W, Chonan T, et al. Effects of submental electrical stimulation during sleep on upper airway patency in patients with obstructive sleep apnea. Am Rev Respir Dis 1989;140:1285–9.
163. Schwartz AR, Thut DC, Russ B, et al. Effect of electrical stimulation of the hypoglossal nerve on airflow mechnaics in the isolated upper airway. Am Rev Respir Dis 1993;147:1144–50.
164. Eisele DW, Smith PL, Alam DSS, et al. Direct hypoglossal nerve stimulation in obstructive sleep apnea. Arch Otolaryngol Head Neck Surg 1997;123:57–61.
165. Servais JJ, Hörmann K, Wallhäusser-Franke E. Unilateral cochlear implantation reduces tinnitus loudness in bimodal hearing: a prospective Study. Front Neurol 2017;8:60.
166. House LR. Cochlear implant: the beginning. Laryngoscope 1987;97:996–7.
167. House WF, Urban J. Long terms results of electrode implantation and electronic stimulation of the cochlea in man. Ann Otol Rhinol Laryngol 1973;82(4):504–17.
168. Mudry A, Mills M. The early history of the cochlear implant. JAMA Otolaryngol Head Neck Surg 2013;139(5):446–53.
169. Eisenberg L, House WF. Initial experience with the cochlear implant in children. Ann Otol Rhinol Laryngol Suppl 1982;91:67–73.
170. Berliner K, Luxford W, House WF. Cochlear implants: 1981-1985. Am J Otol 1985;6:173–86.
171. Edgerton BJ, House WF, Hitselberger W. Hearing by cochlear nucleus stimulation in humans. Ann Otol Rhinol Laryngol Suppl 1982;91:117–24.
172. Schwartz AR, Bennett ML, Smith PL, et al. Therapeutic electrical stimulation of the hypoglossal nerve in obstructive sleep apnea. Arch Otolaryngol Head Neck Surg 2001;127(10):1216–23.
173. Strollo PJ Jr, Soose RJ, Maurer JT, et al. Upper-airway stimulation for obstructive sleep apnea. N Engl J Med 2014;370:139.
174. Woodson BT, Strohl KP, Soose RJ, et al. Upper airway stimulation for obstructive sleep apnea: 5-year outcomes. Otolaryngol Head Neck Surg 2018;159(1):194–202.

The Ethics of Cranial Nerve Implants

Sven Ove Hansson, PhD[a,b],*

KEYWORDS

- Auditory brainstem implant • Cochlear implant • Cranial nerve implant • Ethics
- Explantation • Hypoglossal nerve stimulation • Informed consent
- Vagus nerve stimulation

KEY POINTS

- A large number of the patients who need a cochlear implant do not receive it. This is largely due to socioeconomic and ethnic inequities, which urgently need to be addressed.
- Simpler and cheaper cochlear implants need to be developed for use in developing countries.
- Undesired psychological effects of implants should be taken seriously. They should be evaluated with a strong focus on a patient's own experiences, also in cases of limited communication abilities.
- Informed consent is particularly important for irreversible interventions, such as implants that cannot be removed without considerable risks or other disadvantages. Guidelines should be developed for elective explantation of neuroprosthetic devices.
- Security against unauthorized reprogramming or information harvesting should be a basic technical requirement for all implanted medical devices.

INTRODUCTION

Most cranial nerve implants provide either essential sensory channels to the outer world (sound, balance, vision, and smell) or other functions that are central to social lives (voice, mood, and sleep). The close connection with social communication and personal functioning makes it particularly important to pay attention to an individual patient's expectations, experiences, wishes, and social situation (**Box 1**).

ETHICAL CONSIDERATIONS FOR THE INDIVIDUAL
Informed Consent

A patient's informed consent is a crucial precondition for implant surgery. For consent to be informed, the patient must have a realistic picture of the expected effects of the

Disclosures: Funding: Swedish Research Council, grant 2014-07483. Conflicts of interest: None.
[a] Division of Philosophy, Royal Institute of Technology (KTH), Teknikringen 76, Stockholm 100 44, Sweden; [b] Department of Learning, Informatics, Management and Ethics, Karolinska Institutet, Sweden
* Division of Philosophy, KTH, Teknikringen 76, Stockholm 100 44, Sweden.
E-mail address: soh@kht.se

Box 1
Summary of ethical considerations for implantable stimulators

Ethical considerations for the individual
• Informed consent
• Risks of implantation
• Explantation considerations
• Effects on personality and personal identity
• Implantation for enhancement

Ethical considerations for society
• Distributional issues
• Cultural effects

Ethical considerations of implant research

---

intervention, the potential risks and side effects, and the training and rehabilitation that may be needed. To give consent, a patient must have the required decision-making capacity. That capacity is task specific, and a patient may have it even if decision-making is limited in other contexts, for instance, by a psychiatric condition.[1]

Pediatric patients should be informed and their autonomy respected, although their guardians have the final say. There is evidence that treatment outcomes can be improved if a child patient is actively involved and listened to.[2]

Risks from Receiving Implants

According to the standard view in medical ethics, informed consent (when obtainable) is a necessary but not sufficient condition for any medical intervention. A reasonably favorable risk-benefit assessment is an independent and necessary requirement the intervention to be ethically acceptable. It is a violation of medical ethics to inflict harm that cannot be justified by outweighing medical benefits, even if a patient consents or perhaps even asks for it. A patient desperately looking for a last resort treatment may be willing to undergo an intervention incurring risks that cannot be medically justified and, therefore, should not be offered or performed.

Complications from cochlear implants are now relatively rare, but careful attention is still needed to potential unusual complications.[3] Due to improved technology, there is a tendency to relax audiological criteria, which means that patients may have more to lose in case of a failed intervention. If the expected amelioration in a patient's everyday life is not large enough, then it may not be worth the risk of complications and/or failure of the intervention.[4]

An auditory brainstem implant (ABI) requires a more invasive and complex surgery than a cochlear implant, and the outcome is also clearly inferior to that of a cochlear implant. In addition, there are risks of nonauditory effects of the stimulation of the brainstem, due to effects on structures close to the cochlear nucleus.[5] For patients with no remaining functionality of the acoustic nerve, the benefits of an ABI usually outweigh the risks. For patients with residual functionality of the auditory nerve, however, the choice between a cochlear implant and an ABI has to be based on thorough consideration not only of the expected benefits but also of the potential risks of the two operations.

Vestibular implantation requires an unusually difficult surgery, with a significant risk of causing deafness in hearing patients. There also may be risks of facial nerve paralysis. These implants are still at an experimental stage, and the practice is to perform such operations only on deaf ears, typically in patients who at the same time are receiving a cochlear implant.[6,7] A considerable improvement and validation of surgical techniques seems be needed before these implants are ready for routine clinical use.

The implantation of stimulators in surgically more accessible structures, such as the vagus and hypoglossal nerves, has less problematic risk-benefit assessments. Although vagus nerve implantation is considered relatively safe, there are risks of surgical wound infections, damage to the nerve, and (usually temporary) side effects, such as voice alteration, neck pain, paresthesia, palpitations, and so forth. Patients also may need to have the stimulator turned off in connection with magnetic resonance imaging.[8] Patients should be informed of risks and side effects before the implantation, as part of the basis for informed consent.

The security of neuroimplants has received increased attention due to heightened vigilance against terrorism. Programmable devices can be subject to unauthorized reprogramming, intended to harm the patient. Wireless reprogramming, which is highly convenient in the clinic, makes such attacks easier to perform. This problem has mostly been discussed in connection with cardiac pacemakers and implantable defibrillators,[9] but security against unauthorized manipulations should be a basic technical requirement on all implanted medical devices. Manufacturers should also make sure that a patient's privacy cannot be threatened by surreptitious (wireless) hacking of electronic memories in implants.

Explantation

Although neuroimplants are usually intended for lifelong service, technical malfunction or severe side effects can make removal imperative. If technological development has made an implant outmoded, the question also may arise of replacing a still functioning device by a new one. Close attention must then be paid to the risk of ending up in worse functionality rather than the intended improvement. For cochlear implants, a judicious solution often is possible: if the patient has an implant in only one ear, and implantation in the other ear is possible, then that is an obvious option. Similarly, if the patient has functioning implants in both ears, then replacement by new technology in only one of them may be a reasonable option from a risk-benefit point of view.[10]

Another potential reason for explantation is a recall by the manufacturer. Recalled devices should not be implanted. On the other hand, there are strong reasons not to explant a recalled device as long as it functions well. Patients whose device has been recalled should be informed, however, of the situation so that they can prepare mentally for the increased risk of a need for replacement.[10]

Elective explantation of a functioning implant can be a problematic intervention. On the 1 hand, a decision-competent patient has the right not only to decline an offered treatment but also to end a treatment, even if there are reasons to believe that the medical or social condition will worsen as a result of doing so. For instance, a patient is in her own right to discontinue an ongoing treatment of a laryngeal cancer even if chances of survival will then decrease substantially. In analogy, it could be claimed that a patient is in her right to have her implant removed, if she so wishes. This is highly problematic, however, if an explantation is expected to put her in a significantly worse situation than if she had never received the implant. The total effect of the surgeon's two interventions (implantation + explantation) will then be to worsen the patient's health status. This is contrary to the nonmaleficence requirement of medical ethics, which is not overridden by a patient's wish for a harmful intervention. There is, therefore, a conflict between autonomy and nonmaleficence.

A case reported by Owoc and coworkers[11] illustrates these difficulties. A patient with a unilateral cochlear implant asked to have her implant, including the electrode array at the cochlea, removed, largely in order to connect fully with Deaf culture.

She was not satisfied with deactivation or partial removal. The otologist informed her that later reimplantation would not be possible. Postexplantation ossification at the site of cochleostomy would prevent reimplantation in the same ear, and the nonimplanted ear was already too ossified for implantation. The option of introducing an intracochlear spacer to prevent ossification was rejected by the patient. In the end, after several discussions with the patient, the otologist agreed to remove the implant.

This was no doubt a difficult decision, and presumably the otologist's decision might have been different, for instance, for a high-risk surgical patient. Surgically more complex explantations, such as those of brainstem or vestibular implants, also are more problematic. It can be learned from this case that before implantation, patients should be told of the difficulty and, when applicable, the potential infeasibility of explantation. Owoc and coworkers proposed the creation of "specific CI explantation guidelines to assist in clinical decision-making and patient counseling and education."[11] This is much to be recommended, preferably with an extension to also cover other neuroprosthetic devices.

Effects on Personality and Personal Identity

Medical treatments often have psychological effects, that is, they change a patient's behavior, attitudes, and emotions. In many, hopefully most, cases, these are desirable changes that follow from the restoration of health. In other cases, they are undesired side effects of the treatment. If the psychological changes are large, they may be described as a change in personality. For instance, the psychological effects of Parkinson disease often are characterized as changes in personality.

A person's mental state depends largely on bodily experiences and communications with others. Therefore, medical treatment that restores or substitutes sensory impressions can have considerable psychological effects, as evidenced by the effects of cochlear implants. Because olfactory loss is associated with depression, schizophrenia, and cognitive impairment,[12] studies of the psychological effects of olfactory implants are of considerable interest. Restored ability to speak can have large impacts on a patient's social interactions and relations. All this makes psychological effects of treatments a major concern for otorhinolaryngologists.

The distinction between personality changes and psychological effects that do not change a person's personality is nebulous and not necessarily important for clinical judgments. The term, personality change, usually refers to behavioral changes that are easily noted by others, such as sudden changes in irritability. Evaluations of psychological treatment effects should focus on the patient's own experiences, even if communication abilities are limited. In difficult cases, psychological expertise should be consulted.

Changes in personal identity can be conceived as the third and highest stage on a scale with psychological effects on the first level and personality changes on the second. Ethicists have questioned whether a treatment can at all be acceptable if it leads to a change in personal identity. Should the cognitive abilities of a demented patient be improved at the price that she will not be the same person anymore?

The notion of personal identity, however, is difficult to operationalize for clinical purposes, not least due to the tension between the academic conception of identity as a binary concept and the everyday concept of becoming another person. A Swiss patient who received a brain implant for his Parkinson disease reported that "after the implantation of the permanent needles I became a new person. I knew who I was and where I was again. Strange symptoms and fatigue disappeared. I noticed the difference between past and present quite distinctly."[13] As this example shows, changes that make someone feel like another person need not be undesirable.

In conclusion, when evaluating psychological treatment effects, it is just as important as for somatic symptoms to be specific and to have a strong focus on a patient's own perspective. Sweeping statements about "a new personality" or becoming "another person" should not be taken at face value as reasons to change or refrain from treatment.

ETHICAL CONSIDERATIONS FOR SOCIETY
Distributional Issues

Like other therapeutic interventions, cranial nerve implants typically further social equality, because they improve the social situation of people who are underprivileged due to disease. For instance, cochlear implants improve the living conditions of deaf people, and a similar case can be made for the other cranial nerve implants. The extent of this positive effect depends, however, to a large degree, on the socioeconomic outreach of the intervention. In many countries there are large differences between socioeconomic and ethnic groups in terms of actual implantation. A study based on data from the United States in 1997 showed that children living in low-income areas were less likely to receive a cochlear implant. The investigators of this study defined the "relative rate of implantation" as "the proportion of children who received cochlear implants divided by the proportion of children with severe to profound SNHL [sensorineural hearing loss]". This rate was 1.00 in white children, 0.93 in Asian children, 0.28 in Hispanic children, and 0.10 in black children.[14] According to a study based on the US census in the year 2000, only 55% of the children who were eligible for a cochlear implant actually received it.[15] A later study showed decreased socioeconomic inequalities but persistent large ethnic differences. Still in 2012, black and Hispanic children had only half the ratio of implantation that white and Asian children had.[16] Among those receiving an implant, children in lower-income households have a higher rate of postoperative complications, worse follow-up compliance, and lower rates of sequential bilateral implantation.[17] There also is evidence that postlingually deaf patients with low socioeconomic status have lower chances of receiving an implant than those with higher socioeconomic status.[17]

In order to make sure that all children who need a cochlear implant also receive it, it is necessary to have universal hearing screening of newborns (which is already in place in most developed countries), full funding of the intervention (which in practice requires public funding), and well-organized clinics with the resources needed to perform the interventions. These are issues for political decision makers, but physicians have a key role in showing the need for this intervention, its cost-efficiency, and the large difference it can make for patients and their participation in society. In situations with insufficient resources, physicians are left with the impossible task to achieve "the fair allocation of a limited number of cochlear implants to increasing numbers of potential recipients."[18] Westerberg[18] shows that this problem, as it presents itself in a center for adult patients, can be approached with much the same procedures as for organ transplantation. His deliberations also show, however, that it is much easier to compile a long list of factors that should have no influence than to identify factors that should contribute considerably to priority setting.

There also are large differences between countries in the use of cochlear implants. A recent study reported that in Australia, 98% of the candidate children up to the age of 2 receive an implant, in Sweden and the United Kingdom above 90%, in Germany 65%, and in the United States approximately 50% (with considerable differences between states). In all these countries, at least 90% of all newborn children are screened for hearing loss. The low rate in the United States was attributed to the in-surance system and insufficient referrals and that in Germany to counseling issues. In all these countries, even Australia with its high pediatric utilization, adult utilization is below 10%. Plausible causes of this are the lack of hearing screening in adults, insufficient knowledge in primary care, overly stringent candidacy criteria, and lack of resources.[19] Access to cochlear implants is still severely limited in many developing countries.[20] As noted by Fagan and Tarabichi, a combination of ethical concerns and practical challenges has to be addressed in these countries: "prioritization of cochlear implants when access to hearing aids is limited; patient selection criteria in indigent populations; and lack of availability of simpler, cheaper cochlear implants for indigent patients."[21] The last-mentioned of these concerns is also an issue of corporate social responsibility for the medical technology industry.

Much less information is available about access to other cranial nerve implants. It has been observed, however, that lack of insurance coverage often prevents patients from receiving vagus nerve stimulation against treatment-resistant depression,[22] and similar problems have been reported for hypoglossal nerve implants against obstruc-tive sleep apnea.[23] There is a need for more studies of patients' actual access to medi-cally indicated cranial nerve implants. If deficiencies are identified, countermeasures may have to include improved insurance coverage but also other measures, such as those disucssed in Chang and colleagues'[17] study of inequities in pediatric cochlear implantation: "more intensive training and education; social support ser-vices, especially to single-parent families; automated telephone calls for more frequent follow-up checks; or more hands-on, longitudinal care, such as the suc-cesses detailed in the literature for diabetes mellitus care."

Cultural Effects

Medical treatments can have considerable effects on a patient's social interactions. When many people are affected, this can have widespread effects, affecting what is called (somewhat vaguely) the "culture" of a society. For instance, the introduction of female contraception had large effects on reproduction and gender relations, and antiretroviral human immunodeficiency virus therapy has radically improved condi-tions of life in the subcommunities most affected by that disease.

Several of the treatments based on cranial nerve implants can have a large impact on a patient's life. This applies not least to cochlear implants, both in children and (postlingually operated) adults. As noted by Teagle, there are "few examples of life-changing technology that rival the profound impact that cochlear implant technology has had on children with severe to profound hearing loss."[24] This can be seen not least from their educational and and occupational achievements. Even for children with multiple medical conditions that lessen their chances of developing a spoken lan-guage, perception of environmental sound can make life much easier. For postlin-gually implanted adults, cochlear implants have the important consequences of "increased speech comprehension without visual support, control of their own voice and clearer speech production, less dependence on third parties, increased safety and interaction in conversation and activities, better performance in the work-place and in academic learning, telephone use, and appreciation of music and other entertainment."[25] Thus, both groups gain much in terms of social inclusion and access to cultural activities and assets.

But there is also another perspective. Deaf communities have built up impressive subcultures all over the world, including rich and complex sign languages.[26] These are unique, tightly knit subcultures. In comparison, there is no corresponding Blind culture, possibly because there is no language for the blind, only tactile alphabets, such as Braille, for writing common languages.[27] Contrary to other subcultures, Deaf culture usually is not transmitted from parents to children, but instead "passed on in residential schools, in which Sign is the first language and in which new generations are acculturated."[28] Approximately 96% of all deaf children are born of two hearing parents.[29] Almost all of these parents want their children to hear, and they are, therefore, positive to cochlear implantation. Furthermore, studies indicate that less than 10% of culturally deaf parents in the United States would prefer to have a deaf child.[30] These numbers would seem to guarantee the rapid diminution and ultimate demise of Deaf culture, and understandably some of its proponents have argued for measures that would prevent this from happening.[31] This led to a clash with the medical profession's view of deafness as a disease in need of treatment. With time, however, this conflict has largely abated. A major reason for this is that the usefulness for implanted children of learning sign language has been widely recognized, also among hearing parents.[32,33] Children with implants have often developed a sense of belonging to Deaf culture, whose resistance to implantation has also gradually receded. It now seems plausible that Deaf culture and sign language will survive, albeit (like other subcultures) in modified form and with new relations to the surrounding society.

Every child who can be helped with a cochlear implant should have that opportunity. As discussed above, the major obstacles that prevent this from happening are economic and organizational in nature. There is also a small minority of (almost always deaf) parents who do not wish their child to receive a cochlear implant. The question has been raised whether, in view of the large advantages of implantation in early childhood, parents should be allowed to restrict their child's future life chances by declining the offer of an implant.[34,35] This is part of much larger legal and political issues, concerning the rights of guardians and the criteria for government intervention in families. In jurisdictions that allow parents to make these choices for their children, the physician's role is to respectfully provide these parents with the best possible information about the implant and its impact on the child's future.

Effects of Implants for Enhancement

Neuroimplants have been a major topic in discussions on human enhancement, that is, improvements of the human body that go beyond restoration from disease. Cranial nerve implants can in principle be used to convey signals that a normal human cannot perceive, such as ultrasound or infrasound, infrared or ultraviolet light, magnetic fields, or otherwise odorless chemicals. Much of these discussions has little clinical relevance. There is a small subculture of so-called grinders (body hackers), however, who experiment with modifications on their own bodies. For instance, one person had a magnet implanted in his tragus as part of a loudspeaker system.[36] The implantation was made by a so-called body modification artist (which seems to be a euphemism for quack surgeon). There may be people willing for instance to forgo normal hearing in one ear in order to have a cochlear implant programmed for infrasound or ultrasound. Any contributions of such endeavors would go against the fundamental dictum "first, do not harm" of medical ethics.

The situation is different for patients who already have a cochlear implant. The frequency range is programmable, and the device can in principle be temporarily reset for instance to sounds outside of the normal hearing range. The same applies to hearing aids. Both these types of devices can now be connected with Bluetooth. This facilitates the use of telephones and other external devices as well as listening to a teacher (wearing a microphone) in a noisy classroom. Enhancing applications, such as perception of ultrasound and infrasound, therefore, are possible, with no need for body hacking.

RESEARCH ETHICS

The whole range of general issues in research ethics applies to research on cranial nerve implants. The area has seen a case of unreported conflict of interest, when an article on vagus nerve stimulation was published without a statement acknowledging that all the investigators had financial ties to a company producing a device for this intervention.[37]

In neuroimplantation, studies on animal models usually are required before tests on humans are ethically defensible. Animal experiments are in themselves, however, ethically problematic. The standard 3R concept should be applied: reduce the need for animal experiments as much as possible, refine the experiments to minimize animal suffering, and whenever possible replace animal models for instance by in vitro studies or mathematical simulations.[38] It is also generally agreed that experiments on primates should be avoided as far as possible. This cannot always be achieved in studies of complex functions of the central nervous system. Following the 3R principles then is particularly important.

The recruitment of human subjects for trials of retinal implants has been subject to an extensive discussion, from which much can be learned. Due to the limited kind of light perception that can currently be achieved, few blind persons have been willing to volunteer for trials. It also has been reported that those willing to participate have largely been driven by problematic motives, such as unrealistic hopes about the type of vision they would obtain (a therapeutic misconception)[39] or a wish to make amends for genetically passing on retinitis pigmentosa to their children.[40] Detailed interviews with willing subjects have shown, however, that on closer inspection, their motivations may be less problematic than what has often been assumed. In particular, some blind people consider even rudimentary perception of light as important for their everyday lives, for instance by making them able to "see a doorway" or "avoid a coffee table."[40]

One major retinal implantation project was based in the United States but had the surgery performed in European countries with less stringent ethical requirements on clinical trials than those of the Food and Drug Administration. Preoperation and postoperation procedures took place in the United States. Patients had to pay between $54,000 and $200,000 for being subjects in these experiments.[40] This organization of the trial seems to have fostered and exploited the therapeutic misconception, which should instead have been actively discouraged. Furthermore, the appropriate response to a denied ethical approval is usually to improve the research design, rather than to search for a country with a more permissive legislation.

Many clinical trials with cranial nerve implants can potentially have a large impact on the subjects' future lives, in particular if explantation is risky or perhaps in practice impossible, which makes the trial in reality lifelong. For such trials, the consent procedure should include repeated detailed conversations with the patient, to make sure that the patient understands the trial and its potential effects on her life, and also that the research team understands the subject's motives and grounds for participation.

REFERENCES

1. Christopher PP, Dunn LB. Risk and consent in neuropsychiatric deep brain stimulation: An exemplary analysis of treatment-resistant depression,

obsessive-compulsive disorder, and dementia. In: Clausen J, Levy N, editors. Handbook of neuroethics. Dordrecht: Springer; 2015. p. 589–605.
2. McCabe MA. Involving children and adolescents in medical decision-making: developmental and clinical considerations. J Pediatr Psychol 1996;21:505–16.
3. Shinghal T, et al. Seizure activity following cochlear implantation: Is it the implant? Int J Pediatr Otorhinolaryngol 2012;76:704–7.
4. Mäki-Torkko EM, et al. From isolation and dependence to autonomy – expectations before and experiences after cochlear implantation in adult cochlear implant users and their significant others. Disabil Rehabil 2015;37:541–7.
5. Eisenberg LS, et al. Early communication development of children with auditory brainstem implants. J Deaf Stud Deaf Educ 2018;23:249–60.
6. Poppendieck W, et al. Ethical issues in the development of a vestibular prosthesis. Conf Proc IEEE Eng Med Biol Soc 2011;2011:2265–8.
7. Fornos AP, et al. The vestibular implant: a probe in orbit around the human balance system. J Vestib Res 2017;27:51–61.
8. Jotterand F, et al. Ethics and informed consent of vagus nerve stimulation (VNS) for patients with treatment-resistant depression (TRD). Neuroethics 2010;3: 13–22.
9. Halperin D, et al. Pacemakers and implantable cardiac defibrillators: software radio attacks and zero-power defenses. Proc IEEE Symp Secur Priv 2008;129–42.
10. McCormick TR. Ethical conflicts in caring for patients with cochlear implants. Otol Neurotol 2010;31:1184–9.
11. Owoc MS, et al. Medical and bioethical considerations in elective cochlear implant array removal. J Med Ethics 2018;44:174–9.
12. Ekström I, et al. Smell loss predicts mortality risk regardless of dementia conversion. J Am Geriatr Soc 2017;65:1238–43.
13. Available at: https://alternativeparkinson.com/conquering-alzheimers-with-permanent-needle/. Accessed March 31, 2019.
14. Stern RE, et al. Recent epidemiology of pediatric cochlear implantation in the United States: disparity among children of different ethnic and socioeconomic status. Laryngoscope 2005;115:125–31.
15. Bradham T, Jones J. Cochlear implant candidacy in the United States: prevalence in children 12 months to 6 years of age. Int J Pediatr Otorhinolaryngol 2008;72:1023–8.
16. Tampio AJF, et al. Trends in sociodemographic disparities of pediatric cochlear implantation over a 15-year period. Int J Pediatr Otorhinolaryngol 2018;115: 165–70.
17. Chang DT, et al. Lack of financial barriers to pediatric cochlear implantation: impact of socioeconomic status on access and outcomes. Arch Otolaryngol Head Neck Surg 2010;136:648–57.
18. Westerberg BD. Ethical considerations in resource allocation in a cochlear implant program. J Otolaryngol Head Neck Surg 2008;37:250–5.
19. Sorkin DL, Buchman CA. Cochlear implant access in six developed countries. Otol Neurotol 2016;37:e161–4.
20. Rapport F, et al. Qualitative, multimethod study of behavioural and attitudinal responses to cochlear implantation from the patient and healthcare professional perspective in Australia and the UK: study protocol. BMJ Open 2018;8:e019623.
21. Fagan JJ, Tarabichi M. Cochlear implants in developing countries: practical and ethical considerations. Curr Opin Otolaryngol Head Neck Surg 2018;26:188–9.
22. Bewernick B, Schlaepfer TE. Update on neuromodulation for treatment-resistant depression. F1000Res 2015;4 [pii:F1000 Faculty Rev-1389].

23. Weeks B, et al. Hypoglossal Nerve Stimulator Implantation in a Non-Academic Setting: Two-Year Result. Laryngoscope Investig Otolaryngol 2018;3:315–8.
24. Teagle HFB. Cochlear implantation for children: opening doors to opportunity. J Child Neurol 2012;27:824–6.
25. Vieira SDS, et al. Effects of cochlear implantation on adulthood. Codas 2018; 30:1–8.
26. Kusters A, De Meulder M. Understanding Deafhood: In search of its meanings. Am Ann Deaf 2013;158:428–38.
27. Weisleder P. No such thing as a "Blind Culture". J Child Neurol 2012;27:819–20.
28. Levy N. Reconsidering cochlear implants: the lessons of Martha's Vineyard. Bioethics 2002;16:134–53.
29. Mitchell RE, Karchmer MA. Chasing the mythical ten percent: parental hearing status of deaf and hard of hearing students in the United States. Sign Lang Stud 2004;4:138–63.
30. Johnston T. In one's own image: Ethics and the reproduction of deafness. J Deaf Stud Deaf Educ 2005;10:426–41.
31. Lane H, Bahan B. Ethics of cochlear implantation in young children: A review and reply from a Deaf-World perspective. Otolaryngol Head Neck Surg 1998;119: 297–313.
32. Zaidman-Zait A. Parenting a child with a cochlear implant: a critical incident study. J Deaf Stud Deaf Educ 2007;12:221–41.
33. Kermit P. Choosing for the child with cochlear implants: a note of precaution. Med Health Care Philos 2010;13:157–67.
34. Byrd S, et al. The right not to hear: the ethics of parental refusal of hearing rehabilitation. Laryngoscope 2011;121:1800–4.
35. Nunes R. Ethical dimension of paediatric cochlear implantation. Theor Med 2001; 22:337–49.
36. Innes E. Who needs headphones? Man has 'speakers' IMPLANTED in his ears so he can listen to music all the time. MailOnline. 2013. Available at: https://www.dailymail.co.uk/sciencetech/article-2352690/Rich-Lee-Man-speakers-IMPLANTED-ears-listen-music-time.html. Accessed March 31, 2019.
37. Holden C. The undisclosed background of a paper on a depression treatment. Science 2006;313(5787):598–9.
38. Russell WMS, Burch RL. The principles of humane experimental technique. London: Methuen; 1959.
39. Xia Y, Ren Q. Ethical considerations for voluntary recruitment of visual prosthesis trials. Sci Eng Ethics 2013;19:1099–106.
40. Lane FJ, et al. Perspectives of optic nerve prostheses. Disabil Rehabil Assist Technol 2016;11:301–9.

Concepts in Neural Stimulation

Electrical and Optical Modulation of the Auditory Pathways

Angela Zhu, MPhil, Ahad A. Qureshi, MD, Elliott D. Kozin, MD, Daniel J. Lee, MD*

KEYWORDS

- Neuroprosthetics • Neural stimulation techniques • Sensory disorders
- Optogenetics

KEY POINTS

- Peripheral and central neural pathways are most commonly stimulated using electrical impulses, a paradigm used in all clinical neuroprostheses, such as cochlear implants and auditory brainstem implants.
- Electrical neuromodulation is limited by current spread and channel cross-talk, restricting the number of independent information channels through which to convey sensory information.
- Optogenetic and infrared stimulation are newer neural stimulation techniques that have been used in research to modulate responses both in vitro and in vivo, including the auditory system.
- Novel optogenetics-driven devices may address the shortcomings of electrical stimulation by improving the spatial selectivity of neuron activation.
- Newer neuromodulatory techniques may ultimately lead to better outcomes in patients who must learn to interpret sensory signals through neural stimulation.

INTRODUCTION

Neurons comprise the basic functional unit of the brain and nervous system. Control of neural activity requires understanding the different types of stimuli to which neurons are responsive. Centrally located neurons, such as those of cranial nerves, can be

Disclosures: Dr. Lee received funds from The Bertarelli Foundation (DoD NF170090), Synergia (Swiss National Science Foundation). Rest of the authors do not have any financial conflicts of interest to disclose.
Department of Otolaryngology, Massachusetts Eye and Ear Infirmary, Harvard Medical School, 243 Charles Street, Boston, MA 02114, USA
* Corresponding:
E-mail address: daniel_lee@meei.harvard.edu

triggered by a multitude of stimuli, such as light, chemicals, and pressure. When native neuron function is compromised, interventions to artificially modulate neural activity can improve the arising cranial nerve deficits. Modern clinical neural stimulators are based on electricity, which use electrodes placed in close proximity of neurons that deliver electrical impulses in lieu of normal input signals. Artificial stimulation can restore or supplement function of the nervous system and provide therapy for a variety of sensory disorders.

Clinical neural stimulation is achieved through devices called neuroprosthetics. Neuroprosthetic devices have evolved and improved over the past 50 years, and there have been significant advances in both invasive and noninvasive neural stimulation therapies. Neuroprosthetic devices require some degree of residual nerve activity, and work by bypassing nonfunctional nerve activity loss from trauma or disease. By stimulating second-order or third-order neurons found downstream along the neural pathways, some degree of function can be restored. Hearing loss is a disorder in which neuroprosthetic devices have been heavily used and have been remarkably successful. Hearing loss is one of the most pervasive sensory disorders worldwide, with an estimated 466 million people in the world having disabling hearing loss.[1] For patients with profound hearing loss, auditory implants such as cochlear implants and auditory brainstem implants can provide meaningful sound sensations to most users.[2,3]

Cochlear implants (CIs) and auditory brainstem implants (ABIs) have multichannel electrode arrays to deliver electrical impulses to activate the cochlear nerve or cochlear nucleus neurons in the auditory brainstem, respectively. CIs bypass damaged hair cells to activate postsynaptic spiral ganglion neurons, the axons of which make up the cochlear portion of cranial nerve VIII. The cochlear nerve may however be damaged or absent due to a plethora of reasons, such as congenital malformations, which cause cochlear nerve aplasia or hypoplasia, injury or scarring secondary to trauma, meningitis, otosclerosis, or neoplastic processes, such as vestibular schwannomas formation.[4] Patients with damaged or absent cochlear nerves are not candidates for the cochlear implant and may be candidates for the auditory brainstem implant to provide sound sensations.[3] ABIs bypass the peripheral auditory system by directly activating downstream auditory neurons in the cochlear nucleus of the brainstem.[5] The cochlear nucleus receives most of its input from the cochlear nerve where the processing of auditory input begins, and is the first relay station in the brainstem for all sound information from the ear.[6]

Although CIs and ABIs represent significant advances in how electrical stimulation can be translated clinically, more recent work in the basic sciences has introduced the concept of using light to stimulate neurons. Optical stimulation has been proposed as a novel means of modulating neural function in the auditory system, with millisecond precision in some cases.[7-10] Although early efforts to stimulate neurons with light began as early as 1891,[11] use of lasers for neural activation came under way in the past 60 years.[12] Neurons can be irradiated with different optical wavelengths, from infrared to visible-spectra light.[13] Recently, the concept of light-based neural stimulation has been applied clinically, with light-based implants being tested in in vivo animal models of sciatic, spinal cord, and cochlear nerve dysfunction.[14-17] With the advent of smaller and more modular light power sources, such as micro light-emitting diodes, it has become possible to integrate miniature light sources into fully implantable optogenetic devices that are biocompatible with both central and peripheral neural tissue.[18] The current body of research highlights the advantages of optical stimulation over electrical and provides strong evidence that it can overcome the shortcomings of electricity-based implants.

In this article, we discuss the different methods for neural stimulation and review recent research advances in electrical, infrared, and optogenetics-based neuromodulation applications. We also highlight current studies being conducted on light-based stimulation of the cochlear nerve.

ELECTRICAL NEURAL STIMULATION

Using electricity to clinically stimulate nerves was first demonstrated in 1912, when Perthes developed and described the first electrical nerve stimulator.[19] In their current form, neuroprosthetic devices rely solely on electrical impulses to stimulate neurons.[20] Electrodes are placed in direct contact with the nerve, and may be linked by transmitter wires to stimulators worn either outside or inside the body. (1) Intensity and (2) pulse duration are 2 crucial characteristics of electrical impulses that must be considered when activating neurons. Current intensity is a measure of stimulus strength, and is a flow of electrical charges used to depolarize the neuron and evoke a sensory response. In addition, a minimum/threshold pulse duration of the impulse must be delivered to activate the neuron. Using electrical neural stimulators, clinicians can restore some degree of function in nerves damaged due to disease or trauma. By stimulating nerves directly using neuroprosthetic devices, sensory information bypasses native sensory encoding processes and are transmitted directly to the central nervous system.

CIs are considered the most successful and sophisticated neuroprosthetics, and have successfully helped hundreds of thousands of people with severe to profound hearing loss achieve frequency and sound intensity discrimination and recognition of speech.[2] Electrical stimulation of the auditory system was first demonstrated in 1957, when Djourno and Eyries were able to generate sound sensations in a deaf patient.[21] Modern CIs and ABIs now house multichannel electrodes, and have undergone multiple refinements in hardware and software design since the invention of single-electrode device. Improvements in signal processing and speech coding strategies have led to increased effectiveness of these devices for patients. Altering the pattern of electrode activation became possible when multichannel CIs came into use.[22] By doing so, different frequencies of sound information can be conveyed to the user. Similarly, ABIs have multichannel electrodes configured on a rigid paddle, and use the same external component as the cochlear implant.[3] However, auditory outcomes with ABIs are poor compared with the outcomes from CIs.[3]

LIMITATIONS OF ELECTRICAL STIMULATION

Despite the success of the cochlear implant, these devices do not completely restore hearing. Patient outcomes with CIs are variable and there are no standardized markers to predict which patients will achieve good audiological outcomes with the device. The 8 to 20 stimulation channels of these neuroprosthetic devices do not replace the nearly 30,000 spiral ganglion neurons of the inner ear, with each neuron tuned to a specific best frequency.[23] The limited stimulation channels therefore distort the spatial and temporal patterns of neural information conveyed to the brain. Centrally, the auditory cortex must learn to interpret and process this limited information. Therefore, users of these nerve stimulators do not immediately reach peak performance postimplantation and require a period of experience and learning with the device.[24]

In particular, the performance of ABIs lags significantly behind the performance of CIs. Only a minority of auditory brainstem implant users achieve meaningful word recognition, with most users reporting a generalized environmental sound awareness and speech pattern recognition augmented by lip-reading.[25,26] Furthermore, the design of the implant has not changed in decades.[3] Due to the placement in the lateral recess of the fourth ventricle and the rigid paddle where the electrodes are located, the final position of the electrodes and their angle and distance from the cochlear nucleus can vary greatly from patient to patient postoperatively, which influences audiological outcomes.[27] Similar to the cochlear implant, outcomes vary greatly depending on surgical placement, surgeon experience, and postimplantation programming. The tonotopic organization of the cochlear nucleus is also organized from superficial to deep, in contrast to the linear/coiled architecture of the cochlea.[28] This makes activating frequency-dependent neurons with surface electrodes much more difficult in patients with an auditory brainstem implant.

Why electrical neuromodulation fails to achieve good audiologic outcomes in a subset of patients who use cochlear or ABIs is still not well understood. In part, this can be explained by the nonselective nature of electrical stimulation. One reason for the limited spectral resolution of sound information that auditory implants can convey is that the electrical current spreads from the electrode contacts along the cochlea or the cochlear nucleus, which may be further exacerbated by the conductive nature of perilymph and cerebrospinal fluid surrounding the electrodes.[29] As a result, increasing the number of electrodes will not increase the number of independent excitation channels and may worsen adjacent channel cross-talk.[30] For patients using cochlear implant or ABIs, performance using these implants is limited with complex sounds, such as noisy listening environments, use of tonal languages, and perception of music.[31]

Electrical stimulation causes distortions in the *spatial* coding of auditory neurons.[32] This disturbance is worsened because of the tendency of the stimulus current to radially spread outward from the point of electrode contact.[33] This results in channel cross-talk, where a stimulus targeted to one subgroup of neurons also modulates distant neuron subgroups meant to be targeted by a different or adjacent stimulation channel (**Fig. 1**A). Electrical spread limits the number of independent stimulation channels in the cochlear implant to approximately 10.[34] This limits the fidelity of sound representation to the patient using the implant. The activation of competing pathways

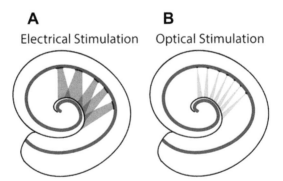

A   **B**
Electrical Stimulation   Optical Stimulation

Fig. 1. Schematic of cochlea showing the spatial selectivity of electrical versus optical activation. (*A*) Electrical activation leads to spread of stimulation current from the electrode point of contact, leading to broad activation of neurons from each electrode. In limited anatomic spaces such as the cochlea, increasing the number of electrode contacts will not help increase the number of independent information channels. (*B*) Optical stimulation enables a greater number of optical contacts. Due to the spatially confined spread of light, the theoretic number of independent information channels can be greatly increased.

can also cause nonauditory side effects, such as dizziness, facial twitching, and pain. One method to improve the spatial selectivity of CIs is to change the electrode configuration. Most implants use monopolar stimulation, which produces broad electric fields and may activate wide tonotopic areas.[35] In monopolar stimulation, there is 1 active electrode, and 1 negative electrode. In bipolar or tripolar stimulation, there are 2 or 3 active electrodes. This allows narrower electric fields to be generated, but at the expense of requiring higher current levels to reach threshold.[35]

The disturbance of electrical stimulation to *temporal*, or time-dependent, coding of sound information stem from the tendency of electricity to recruit nearby auditory neurons with increasing electrical current.[36] The dynamic range, defined as the width of perceptual sound threshold to uncomfortably loud sound, is much narrower in electrical stimulation compared with acoustic hearing, which ranges from 10 to 100 dB.[37] This means that patients using auditory prostheses have a small window through which to adjust their device to render environmental sounds audible but not uncomfortably loud or produce nonauditory side effects. Although modern speech processors use digital algorithms to control the dynamic gain and map stimulus intensity, many patients with CIs require manual adjustment of external speech processor settings.[38] In addition, the narrow dynamic range of electrically driven CIs causes low current intensity "resolution," thereby causing limited speech understanding in noisy environments. A study in cats showed that using penetrating electrodes in the cochlear nerve of cats could improve the temporal transmission of brainstem responses.[39] However, this type of intraneural stimulation is more invasive, and ongoing studies by Hubert H. Lim, Thomas Lenarz, and others will explore the utility of this new approach (**Fig. 1**).

LIGHT-BASED NEUROMODULATION: INFRARED NEURAL STIMULATION

In contrast to electricity, light can be spatially focused. This improvement in spatial selectivity can theoretically increase the number of independent channels that these devices provide (see **Fig. 1B**).[40,41] The auditory periphery may be particularly suited to light-based neuromodulation due to the tonotopic organization of frequency-tuned cochlear neurons. Light can therefore stimulate specific subsets of neurons along the cochlear tonotopic axis to convey frequency information. In the auditory system, this functional increase has the potential to dramatically improve the fidelity of hearing and improve speech perception. Stimulation of cochlear nerves using infrared wavelength light has been studied as a novel neuromodulatory method in the peripheral nervous system as well as in the auditory system.[42,43]

Infrared stimulation works by transiently and locally heating neural tissue.[13] In neurons, this temperature increase causes a capacitive current that depolarizes the neuron cell membrane, causing an action potential.[12] Infrared stimulation was first successfully demonstrated in peripheral motor and sensory neurons.[44] Since then, infrared stimulation of cochlear neurons has been demonstrated in a variety of animal models in the laboratory[43,45,46] using microsecond to millisecond duration pulses.[47] The advantages of infrared stimulation are improved spatial selectivity, minimization of the electrical stimulation artifact, and the ability to deliver stimuli without direct nerve contact. In early studies of cochlear activation using infrared stimulation, it was demonstrated that spectral spread of spiral ganglion neuron activation in infrared-stimulated neurons was similar to that of pure tone acoustic stimulation, and was more narrow than when neurons were stimulated with a monopolar electrode configuration.[45] Unlike optogenetic methods, use of infrared radiation does not require genetic manipulation to render neurons light-sensitive. In addition to peripheral nerves, the safety of infrared stimulation was also demonstrated in the brainstem. In the rat cochlear nucleus, in vivo infrared stimulation of second-order cochlear nucleus neurons produced central auditory responses without evidence of tissue damage.[48]

However, it is unclear whether infrared radiation directly stimulates neurons by causing membrane depolarization and a resulting action potential, or if activation is due to secondary stimuli such as a photoacoustic effect, whereby an acoustic "click" is generated from the rapid expansion of heated water and the resulting pressure wave.[49,50] Another possible mechanism for activation is the creation of a pressure wave that induces hair cell–mediated responses through acoustic artifacts.[51] If hair cell–mediated responses is the main mechanism through which infrared radiation activates neurons, this would be of limited benefit in profoundly deaf patients with nonfunctional or damaged hair cells. In addition, adverse side effects of infrared neural stimulation, such as increased cochlear pressure, have been reported.[51] Furthermore infrared stimulation was able to evoke responses only in animals with some level of residual hearing but failed to evoke responses in deaf animals,[52] or evoked responses only in animals that also responded to acoustic stimuli.[53] In a study of infrared stimulation of the rat cochlear nucleus, which is downstream in the auditory pathways from cochlear hair cells, no responses were measured in the inferior colliculus, the main midbrain auditory nucleus, after lesioning the cochlear nerve at the internal auditory meatus[48] (**Fig. 2**). The elimination of central responses after deafening suggests that the responses produced by infrared stimulation are due to photoacoustic artifact, and has been corroborated in other studies.[54,55] Finally, the high energy requirement

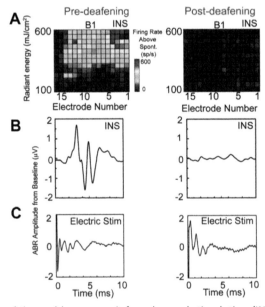

Fig. 2. After lesion of the cochlear nerve, infrared neural stimulation (INS) did not produce detectable midbrain responses. However, electrically evoked responses were still present. (*A*) Inferior colliculus firing responses before and after deafening. (*B*) Auditory brainstem responses (ABRs) after cochlear nucleus infrared stimulation before and after deafening, showing extinction of the response post-deafening. (*C*) ABRs evoked from electrical cochlear nucleus stimulation remained after deafening. (*Adapted from* Verma, Rohit U., et al. "Auditory responses to electric and infrared neural stimulation of the rat cochlear nucleus." Hearing research 310 (2014): 69-75; with permission.)

of infrared radiation per pulse (16–160 μJ) is much greater than what is practical for implantable prostheses and prohibits effective translation of this technology to clinical applications.[56]

LIGHT-BASED NEUROMODULATION: OPTOGENETICS

Optogenetics is the use of visible-spectrum light to control neural activity, and was first developed in 2002 as a powerful neuroscience research tool to study brain circuits in vivo.[57] Using optogenetic technology, it became possible to finely tune neural stimulation with millisecond precision and with a much lower energy requirement than infrared neural stimulation.[58] Furthermore, the optogenetic mechanism of light stimulation is well understood,[57,59] whereas the mechanism of infrared stimulation on neural activation is still unclear.[48] In the presence of visible-spectra light, light-sensitive cell membrane channels known as opsins open to allow the inward flow of cations, causing depolarization of the neuron (**Fig. 3**). These next-generation implants may allow for finer spatial resolution of implants and may enhance perceptual performance.[60]

In contrast to infrared or electrical neural stimulation, optogenetics requires genetic modification of cells to express opsins.[61] These light-activated opsin protein channels called rhodopsins originate in photosensitive algae, and must be expressed in the desired neural cell population in mammalian cells.[57] This has been achieved either through use of transgenic animals, whereby the channelrhodopsin is genetically expressed prenatally, or through use of viral vectors to deliver channelrhodopsins into the genome of a wild-type animal postnatally.[41]

The ideal opsin for neural stimulation in the auditory system would need to have (1) temporal kinetics fast enough to convey speech information, (2) low activation threshold to minimize energy requirements for the neuroprosthesis power source,

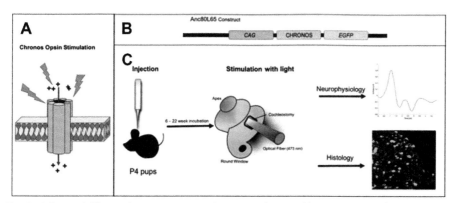

Fig. 3. Schematic illustrating an optogenetic approach to cochlear activation. (*A*) Chronos is an excitatory opsin that allows cations to cross a transmembrane channel after opening to blue (473 nm) light. This depolarizes the neuron. (*B*) Viral vector Anc80L65, which is an ancestral adeno-associated virus, to deliver the Chronos opsin to neurons. CAG is the promoter that drives Chronos expression, and EGFP is the reporter gene that causes green fluorescence. (*C*) Experimental sequence showing 4-day-old (P4) mice injected via round window, then subsequent cochleostomy and insertion of the optical fiber into the proximal basal turn of the cochlea, and further histology and neurophysiology testing. (*From* Duarte, Maria J., et al. "Ancestral adeno-associated virus vector delivery of opsins to spiral ganglion neurons: implications for optogenetic cochlear implants." Molecular Therapy 26.8 (2018): 1931-1939; with permission.)

and (3) have either spiral ganglion neuron or cochlear nucleus neuron selectivity through a specific promoter. One of the first and most well-characterized opsins is known as channelrhodopsin-2 (ChR2).[59] In the auditory system, ChR2-mediated light activation has been successfully demonstrated at several points in the auditory pathway, including at the spiral ganglion neurons,[23,41,62] the cochlear nucleus,[9,63,64] and the inferior colliculus.[10]

A challenge in the translation of optogenetics to clinical applications is the need for fast-activating opsins that can encode auditory information at high stimulation rates. Modern CIs and ABIs are programmed to deliver approximately 250 electrical pulses per second.[33] In contrast, ChR2 cannot follow pulses faster than 60 pulses per second.[65] This challenge has been addressed with the discovery of ultrafast opsins (such as Chronos and ChETA),[61,66,67] as well as mutating amino acid residues in ChR2 to create a greater diversity of excitatory opsins.[68] For example, Chronos is a fast blue-light responsive opsin that can allow neurons to respond to rates of light stimulation up to 448 pulses per second, and is activated at lower thresholds than ChR2.[9] In addition, the kinetics of Chronos can be improved to allow for even higher

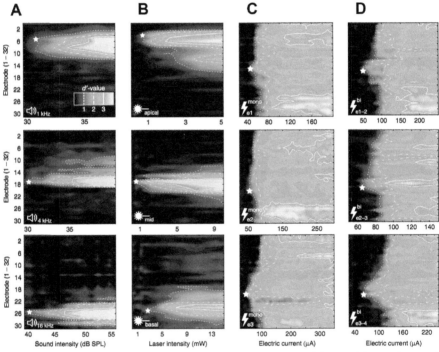

Fig. 4. Spatial tuning curves in gerbil cochleae stimulated with (A) sound (top: 1 kHz, middle: 4 kHz, bottom: 16 kHz), (B) blue (473 nm wavelength) light laser (top: apical turn, middle: middle turn, bottom: basal turn), (C) monopolar electric current (top: electrode 1, middle: electrode 2, bottom: electrode 3), and (D) bipolar electric current (top: electrode 1&2, middle: electrode 2&3, bottom: electrode 3&4). Optogenetic stimulation shows near-physiologic width of spiral ganglion neuron activation compared with pure tone acoustic stimuli. Yellow shows the highest multi-unit neuron firing rate normalized to zero-intensity stimulation (blue). (*From* Dieter, Alexander, et al. "Near physiological spectral selectivity of cochlear optogenetics." *Nature communications* 10 (2019), open access; with permission.)

stimulation rates. Functional expression of Chronos can be further optimized by adding trafficking sequences that target opsin expression to the neuron cell membrane, rather than remaining trapped intracellularly in the Golgi apparatus, where it is less likely that light will elicit an action potential.[69] This optimization technique further enables ultrafast opsin transfer, and may drive stimulation with the high light pulses necessary to convey speech cues.

The goal of successful neural stimulation in the auditory system is to decrease the spread of excitation and therefore improve the frequency and intensity resolution of cochlear implants and ABIs. Improved spatial selectivity of optogenetic activation in the cochlear nerve has been demonstrated to be superior to electrical stimulation in multiple studies using rodent models of the cochlear implant.[8,23,60] Therefore, ChR2-mediated stimulation of the cochlea shows improved frequency resolution and facilitates a larger output dynamic range than electrical stimulation.[67] This has been demonstrated using neurophysiology recordings in the inferior colliculus, a relay nucleus in the central auditory system.[41,60] Optical stimulation was even shown to have comparable physiologic frequency selectivity as auditory stimulation at low light levels, and a much narrower excitation spread in the inferior colliculus than even bipolar electrical stimulation[8] (**Fig. 4**).

The utility of optogenetics to restore sensory deficits is already being tested in human subjects in the visual system.[70,71] Currently, there are ongoing clinical trials investigating the use of adeno-associated viruses with channelrhodopsins to optogenetically restore rudimentary visual sense to patients with retinitis pigmentosa, a degenerative retinal disease with no available treatments that eventually leads to blindness.[72]

SUMMARY

The emergence of novel neuromodulation techniques offer the potential for therapeutic solutions for wide-ranging disorders, such as hearing loss, chronic pain, and other neurologic disorders. Electrical neuromodulation has been the gold standard for rehabilitating sensory disorders but suffers from shortcomings, such as the broad activation of neurons from electrode contacts, overlapping channel interaction, and low dynamic range of sound coding. Optogenetic-mediated neural stimulation has spatial advantages over electrical stimulation, although matching the temporal fidelity of optical stimulation to native auditory signaling still requires further research. There has been substantial progress in light-based neural stimulation, and the potential to improve outcomes for patients using next-generation optical prostheses attests to the importance of understanding the basic physiology behind clinical nerve stimulation.

REFERENCES

1. World Health Organization Media centre. WHO|Deafness and hearing loss. World Health Organization. Available at: entity/mediacentre/factsheets/fs300/en/index.html. Accessed April 29, 2019.
2. Eshraghi AA, Nazarian R, Telischi FF, et al. The cochlear implant: historical aspects and future prospects. Anat Rec 2012. https://doi.org/10.1002/ar.22580.
3. Wong K, Kozin ED, Kanumuri VV, et al. Auditory brainstem implants: recent progress and future perspectives. Front Neurosci 2019. https://doi.org/10.3389/fnins.2019.00010.
4. Kuchta J. Neuroprosthetic hearing with auditory brainstem implants. Biomed Tech 2004. https://doi.org/10.1515/BMT.2004.017.

5. Colletti V, Carner M, Miorelli V, et al. Auditory brainstem implant (ABI): new frontiers in adults and children. Otolaryngol Head Neck Surg 2005. https://doi.org/10.1016/j.otohns.2005.03.022.

6. Shepherd RK, McCreery DB. Basis of electrical stimulation of the cochlea and the cochlear nucleus. Adv Otorhinolaryngol 2006. https://doi.org/10.1159/000094652.

7. Jeschke M, Moser T. Considering optogenetic stimulation for cochlear implants. Hear Res 2015. https://doi.org/10.1016/j.heares.2015.01.005.

8. Dieter A, Duque-Afonso CJ, Rankovic V, et al. Near physiological spectral selectivity of cochlear optogenetics. Nat Commun 2019;10(1):1962.

9. Hight AE, Kozin ED, Darrow K, et al. Superior temporal resolution of Chronos versus channelrhodopsin-2 in an optogenetic model of the auditory brainstem implant. Hear Res 2015. https://doi.org/10.1016/j.heares.2015.01.004.

10. Guo W, Hight AE, Chen JX, et al. Hearing the light: neural and perceptual encoding of optogenetic stimulation in the central auditory pathway. Sci Rep 2015. https://doi.org/10.1038/srep10319.

11. Arsonval AD. La fibre musculaire est directement excitable par la lumiere. C R Soc Biol 1891;43:318–20.

12. Tan X, Rajguru S, Young H, et al. Radiant energy required for infrared neural stimulation. Sci Rep 2015. https://doi.org/10.1038/srep13273.

13. Richter CP, Tan X. Photons and neurons. Hear Res 2014. https://doi.org/10.1016/j.heares.2014.03.008.

14. Montgomery KL, Iyer SM, Christensen AJ, et al. Beyond the brain: optogenetic control in the spinal cord and peripheral nervous system. Sci Transl Med 2016. https://doi.org/10.1126/scitranslmed.aad7577.

15. Montgomery KL, Yeh AJ, Ho JS, et al. Wirelessly powered, fully internal optogenetics for brain, spinal and peripheral circuits in mice. Nat Methods 2015. https://doi.org/10.1038/nmeth.3536.

16. Maimon BE, Sparks K, Srinivasan S, et al. Spectrally distinct channelrhodopsins for two-colour optogenetic peripheral nerve stimulation. Nat Biomed Eng 2018. https://doi.org/10.1038/s41551-018-0255-5.

17. Hernandez Gonzalez VH, Moser T. Optogenetic stimulation for cochlear prosthetics. In: Appasani K, editor. Optogenetics: from neuronal function to mapping and disease biology. Cambridge, UK: Cambridge University Press; 2017. p. 442–52. https://doi.org/10.1017/9781107281875.032.

18. Anikeeva P. Optogenetics unleashed. Nat Biotechnol 2016. https://doi.org/10.1038/nbt.3458.

19. Marhofer P, Harrop-Griffiths W. Nerve location in regional anaesthesia: finding what lies beneath the skin. Br J Anaesth 2011. https://doi.org/10.1093/bja/aeq358.

20. Grill WM, Kirsch RF. Neuroprosthetic applications of electrical stimulation. Assist Technol 2000. https://doi.org/10.1080/10400435.2000.10132006.

21. Eisen MD. Djourno, eyries, and the first implanted electrical neural stimulator to restore hearing. Otol Neurotol 2003. https://doi.org/10.1097/00129492-200305000-00025.

22. Mudry A, Mills M. The early history of the cochlear implant: a retrospective. JAMA Otolaryngol Head Neck Surg 2013. https://doi.org/10.1001/jamaoto.2013.293.

23. Hernandez VH, Gehrt A, Reuter K, et al. Optogenetic stimulation of the auditory pathway. J Clin Invest 2014. https://doi.org/10.1172/JCI69050.

24. Fu QJ, Galvin JJ. Maximizing cochlear implant patients' performance with advanced speech training procedures. Hear Res 2008. https://doi.org/10.1016/j.heares.2007.11.010.

25. Colletti V, Shannon RV. Open set speech perception with auditory brainstem implant? Laryngoscope 2005. https://doi.org/10.1097/01.mlg.0000178327.42926.ec.

26. Noij KS, Kozin ED, Sethi R, et al. Systematic review of nontumor pediatric auditory brainstem implant outcomes. Otolaryngol Head Neck Surg 2015. https://doi.org/10.1177/0194599815596929.

27. Barber SR, Kozin ED, Remenschneider AK, et al. Auditory brainstem implant array position varies widely among adult and pediatric patients and is associated with perception. Ear Hear 2017. https://doi.org/10.1097/AUD.0000000000000448.

28. Deep NL, Choudhury B, Roland JT. Auditory brainstem implantation: an overview. J Neurol Surg B Skull Base 2019. https://doi.org/10.1055/s-0039-1679891.

29. Chen JX, Kozin E, Brown MC, et al. Optogenetics and auditory implants. In: Appasani K, editor. Optogenetics: from neuronal function to mapping and disease biology. Cambridge, UK: Cambridge University Press; 2017. p. 421–41. https://doi.org/10.1017/9781107281875.031.

30. Boëx C, de Balthasar C, Kós M-I, et al. Electrical field interactions in different cochlear implant systems. J Acoust Soc Am 2003. https://doi.org/10.1121/1.1610451.

31. McDermott HJ. Music perception with cochlear implants: a review. Trends Amplif 2004;8(2):49–82.

32. Clark GM. Electrical stimulation of the auditory nerve: the coding of frequency, the perception of pitch and the development of cochlear implant speech processing strategies for profoundly deaf people. Clin Exp Pharmacol Physiol 1996;23(9):766–76.

33. Loizou PC. Introduction to cochlear implants. IEEE Eng Med Biol Mag 1999. https://doi.org/10.1109/51.740962.

34. Middlebrooks JC, Bierer JA, Snyder RL. Cochlear implants: the view from the brain. Curr Opin Neurobiol 2005. https://doi.org/10.1016/j.conb.2005.06.004.

35. Zhu Z, Tang Q, Zeng FG, et al. Cochlear-implant spatial selectivity with monopolar, bipolar and tripolar stimulation. Hear Res 2012. https://doi.org/10.1016/j.heares.2011.11.005.

36. Venail F, Mura T, Akkari M, et al. Modeling of auditory neuron response thresholds with cochlear implants. Biomed Res Int 2015. https://doi.org/10.1155/2015/394687.

37. Kam ACS, Wong LLN. Comparison of performance with wide dynamic range compression and linear amplification. J Am Acad Audiol 1999;10(8):445–57.

38. Zeng FG, Rebscher S, Harrison W, et al. Cochlear implants: system design, integration, and evaluation. IEEE Rev Biomed Eng 2008. https://doi.org/10.1109/RBME.2008.2008250.

39. Middlebrooks JC, Snyder RL. Selective electrical stimulation of the auditory nerve activates a pathway specialized for high temporal acuity. J Neurosci 2010. https://doi.org/10.1523/jneurosci.4949-09.2010.

40. Moser T. Optogenetic stimulation of the auditory pathway for research and future prosthetics. Curr Opin Neurobiol 2015. https://doi.org/10.1016/j.conb.2015.01.004.

41. Duarte MJ, Kanumuri VV, Landegger LD, et al. Ancestral adeno-associated virus vector delivery of opsins to spiral ganglion neurons: implications for optogenetic cochlear implants. Mol Ther 2018. https://doi.org/10.1016/j.ymthe.2018.05.023.

42. Rajguru SM, Richter CP, Matic AI, et al. Infrared photostimulation of the crista ampullaris. J Physiol 2011. https://doi.org/10.1113/jphysiol.2010.198333.

43. Izzo AD, Walsh JT, Jansen ED, et al. Optical parameter variability in laser nerve stimulation: a study of pulse duration, repetition rate, and wavelength. IEEE Trans Biomed Eng 2007. https://doi.org/10.1109/TBME.2007.892925.

44. Duke AR, Cayce JM, Malphrus JD, et al. Combined optical and electrical stimulation of neural tissue in vivo. J Biomed Opt 2009. https://doi.org/10.1117/1.3257230.

45. Richter CP, Rajguru SM, Matic AI, et al. Spread of cochlear excitation during stimulation with pulsed infrared radiation: inferior colliculus measurements. J Neural Eng 2011. https://doi.org/10.1088/1741-2560/8/5/056006.

46. Rajguru SM, Matic AI, Robinson AM, et al. Optical cochlear implants: evaluation of surgical approach and laser parameters in cats. Hear Res 2010. https://doi.org/10.1016/j.heares.2010.06.021.

47. Izzo AD, Richter CP, Jansen ED, et al. Laser stimulation of the auditory nerve. Lasers Surg Med 2006. https://doi.org/10.1002/lsm.20358.

48. Verma RU, Guex AA, Hancock KE, et al. Auditory responses to electric and infrared neural stimulation of the rat cochlear nucleus. Hear Res 2014. https://doi.org/10.1016/j.heares.2014.01.008.

49. Wells J, Kao C, Konrad P, et al. Biophysical mechanisms of transient optical stimulation of peripheral nerve. Biophys J 2007. https://doi.org/10.1529/biophysj.107.104786.

50. Jacques SL. Laser-tissue interactions: photochemical, photothermal, and photomechanical. Surg Clin North Am 1992. https://doi.org/10.1016/S0039-6109(16)45731-2.

51. Teudt IU, Maier H, Richter CP, et al. Acoustic events and "optophonic" cochlear responses induced by pulsed near-infrared LASER. IEEE Trans Biomed Eng 2011. https://doi.org/10.1109/TBME.2011.2108297.

52. Thompson AC, Fallon JB, Wise AK, et al. Infrared neural stimulation fails to evoke neural activity in the deaf guinea pig cochlea. Hear Res 2015. https://doi.org/10.1016/j.heares.2015.03.005.

53. Richter CP, Bayon R, Izzo AD, et al. Optical stimulation of auditory neurons: effects of acute and chronic deafening. Hear Res 2008. https://doi.org/10.1016/j.heares.2008.01.011.

54. Schultz M, Baumhoff P, Maier H, et al. Nanosecond laser pulse stimulation of the inner ear—a wavelength study. Biomed Opt Express 2012. https://doi.org/10.1364/BOE.3.003332.

55. Kallweit N, Baumhoff P, Krueger A, et al. Optoacoustic effect is responsible for laser-induced cochlear responses. Sci Rep 2016. https://doi.org/10.1038/srep28141.

56. Izzo AD, Walsh JT, Ralph H, et al. Laser stimulation of auditory neurons: effect of shorter pulse duration and penetration depth. Biophys J 2008. https://doi.org/10.1529/biophysj.107.117150.

57. Boyden ES, Zhang F, Bamberg E, et al. Millisecond-timescale, genetically targeted optical control of neural activity. Nat Neurosci 2005. https://doi.org/10.1038/nn1525.

58. Dombrowski T, Rankovic V, Moser T. Toward the optical cochlear implant. Cold Spring Harb Perspect Med 2018. https://doi.org/10.1101/cshperspect.a033225.

59. Nagel G, Szellas T, Huhn W, et al. Channelrhodopsin-2, a directly light-gated cation-selective membrane channel. Proc Natl Acad Sci U S A 2003. https://doi.org/10.1073/pnas.1936192100.

60. Wrobel C, Dieter A, Huet A, et al. Optogenetic stimulation of cochlear neurons activates the auditory pathway and restores auditory-driven behavior in deaf adult gerbils. Sci Transl Med 2018. https://doi.org/10.1126/scitranslmed.aao0540.

61. Klapoetke NC, Murata Y, Kim SS, et al. Independent optical excitation of distinct neural populations. Nat Methods 2014. https://doi.org/10.1038/nmeth.2836.
62. Meng X, Hight AE, Kozin ED, et al. Generation of a novel transgenic ChR2 mouse to investigate cochlear implant model based on optogenetics. Otolaryngol Neck Surg 2014. https://doi.org/10.1177/0194599814541627a179.
63. Darrow KN, Slama MCC, Kozin ED, et al. Optogenetic stimulation of the cochlear nucleus using channelrhodopsin-2 evokes activity in the central auditory pathways. Brain Res 2015. https://doi.org/10.1016/j.brainres.2014.11.044.
64. Shimano T, Fyk-Kolodziej B, Mirza N, et al. Assessment of the AAV-mediated expression of channelrhodopsin-2 and halorhodopsin in brainstem neurons mediating auditory signaling. Brain Res 2013. https://doi.org/10.1016/j.brainres.2012.10.030.
65. Berndt A, Schoenenberger P, Mattis J, et al. High-efficiency channelrhodopsins for fast neuronal stimulation at low light levels. Proc Natl Acad Sci U S A 2011. https://doi.org/10.1073/pnas.1017210108.
66. Mager T, Lopez de la Morena D, Senn V, et al. High frequency neural spiking and auditory signaling by ultrafast red-shifted optogenetics. Nat Commun 2018. https://doi.org/10.1038/s41467-018-04146-3.
67. Ronzitti E, Conti R, Zampini V, et al. Submillisecond optogenetic control of neuronal firing with two-photon holographic photoactivation of chronos. J Neurosci 2017. https://doi.org/10.1523/jneurosci.1246-17.2017.
68. Guru A, Post RJ, Ho YY, et al. Making sense of optogenetics. Int J Neuropsychopharmacol 2015. https://doi.org/10.1093/ijnp/pyv079.
69. Keppeler D, Merino RM, Lopez de la Morena D, et al. Ultrafast optogenetic stimulation of the auditory pathway by targeting-optimized Chronos. EMBO J 2018. https://doi.org/10.15252/embj.201899649.
70. ClinicalTrials.gov. RST-001 Phase I/II trail for advanced retinitis pigmentosa. 2015. Available at: https://clinicaltrials.gov/ct2/show/NCT02556736. Accessed May 27, 2019.
71. GenSight Biologics. A phase 1/2a, open-label, non-randomized, dose-escalation study to evaluate the safety and tolerability of GS030 in subjects with retinitis pigmentosa. Bethesda (MD): U.S. National Institute of Health; 2018. Available at: https://clinicaltrials.gov/ct2/show/NCT03326336. Accessed May 27, 2019.
72. Facts about retinitis pigmentosa. Available at: https://nei.nih.gov/health/pigmentosa/pigmentosa_facts. Accessed May 27, 2019.

Central Effects of Cranial Nerve Stimulation

Gavriel D. Kohlberg, MD[a], Ravi N. Samy, MD[b],*

KEYWORDS

- Cortical adaptation • Central reorganization • Vagal nerve stimulation
- Cochlear implant • Central processing • Hearing loss

KEY POINTS

- Vagus (or vagal) nerve stimulation is an approved therapy for epilepsy, depression, and migraine headache.
- Cochlear nerve stimulation through cochlear implantation is used to treat hearing loss ranging from severe to profound. Even those with significant residual hearing can be implanted.
- Chronic stimulation of the vagus and cochlear nerves lead to reorganization of cortical processes.

PURPOSE OF REVIEW

This article reviews the current literature on cranial nerve stimulation for the purpose of achieving therapeutic effects via altering central nervous system activity. Vagus nerve stimulation (VNS) has been extensively studied and approved for treatment of epilepsy. More recently, VNS has been approved for treatment of depression and headache. Trigeminal nerve stimulation has also been approved for treatment of headache. Cochlear nerve stimulation via cochlear implant (CI) alters brain activity for the purpose of increased sound and speech perception. Many other indications related to central effects of cranial nerve stimulation are actively being explored. Yet the mechanism of action of each of central effects of cranial nerve stimulation for all indications remains incompletely elucidated. Further research on both mechanisms and indications of

Disclosure Statement: G.D. Kohlberg: Research funding from Cochlear Corporation. R.N. Samy: Research funding and consultant for Cochlear Corporation.
[a] Division of Otology and Neurotology, Department of Otolaryngology – Head and Neck Surgery, University of Washington School of Medicine, 1959 NE Pacific Street, Box 356161, Seattle, WA 98195 – 6161, USA; [b] Division of Otology/Neurotology, Neurotology Fellowship, Department of Otolaryngology – Head and Neck Surgery, University of Cincinnati College of Medicine, Neurosensory Disorders Center at University of Cincinnati Gardner Neuroscience Institute, Cincinnati Children's Hospital Medical Center, 213 Albert Sabin, Way, MSB 6009C, Cincinnati, OH 45267-0528, USA
* Corresponding author.
E-mail address: ravi.samy@uc.edu
Twitter: @CISurgeon (R.N.S.)

central effects of cranial nerve stimulation has the potential to alleviate burden of disease in a large array of conditions.

INTRODUCTION

Although the stimulation of cranial nerves is often considered as a therapy for dysfunction of the peripheral component of the nerve of interest, several cranial nerve stimulators are known to have considerable impact on the central nervous system (CNS) and have been examined specifically for their central effects. The 2 most well-known examples of this are vagal nerve stimulation (VNS) for treatment of epilepsy and cochlear nerve stimulation for hearing loss. Additional indications for cranial nerve stimulation, specifically for the central effects of the stimulation, exist and devices are available commercially. Because of the well-recognized central effects, potential to expand indications are being actively investigated. Despite the enthusiasm to expand indications, the mechanisms of action are not well understood. Complex neural networks and interconnections exist **(Fig. 1** – will need to request permission to reprint) that make elucidating the exact mechanism of these effects challenging to understand. In this article, we introduce the concept that peripheral stimulation of cranial nerves induces central changes that play a role in the underlying effects of these stimulators. We specifically review the most well-studied implantable stimulators in the

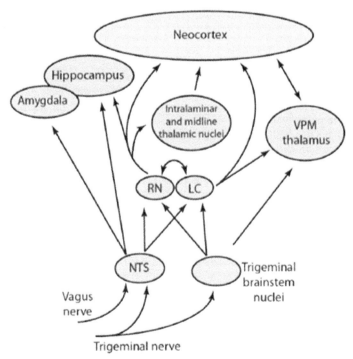

Fig. 1. Central mechanisms of vagal nerve and TNS. Peripheral stimulation of the vagus and trigeminal nerves has effect on the CNS via ascending projections. These interactions represent an incomplete depiction of the complex pathways that alter the CNS activity with peripheral neural stimulation. LC, locus coeruleus; RN, raphe nuclei; VPM, ventral posterior medial thalamus. (*From* Fanselow E. Central Mechanisms of Cranial Nerve Stimulation from Epilepsy. Surg Neurol Int. 2012; 3(Suppl 4): S247–S254; with permission.)

VNS and cochlear implant (CI). However, this concept of centrally induced changes may apply to many of the emerging cranial nerve stimulators (hypoglossal nerve stimulator, vestibular implant) due to the various interconnections with the CNS.[1,2]

Future work will be necessary to explore these concepts as these devices become more available.

CENTRAL EFFECTS OF VAGUS NERVE STIMULATION

At first glance, it is difficult to understand why a peripheral nerve stimulator like the VNS would be indicated for a central process like epilepsy, depression, or migraine headache. Yet, there is substantial evidence that the VNS is a device with significant benefit in these conditions. It was initially approved for epilepsy, and as the benefit became apparent and the concept of effect on the CNS developed, the applications expanded to include depression and migraine. There are a variety of central changes that take place with stimulation of the vagus nerve, and the specific effect of each of these changes is difficult to quantify. Nonetheless, it is likely that each of these effects contributes somewhat to the mechanism of benefit from VNS in each condition. This section reviews the science underlying the central changes with VNS, and each of the indications for use. It is intended to introduce the potential mechanisms of central changes that take place with peripheral cranial nerve stimulation, and the reader is referred to the references for a more detailed review.

EPILEPSY

The potential for VNS to alter seizure activity was first described in 1952 when Zanchetti and colleagues[3] noted that stimulation of the vagus nerve stopped seizure activity in a chemically induced seizure model of cats. Ultimately, after extensive research, VNS was approved for treatment of refractory epilepsy by the Food and Drug Administration (FDA) in 1997. VNS has been found to reduce the number of seizures by more than 50% in 40% of VNS recipients. As of 2015, more than 100,000 VNS devices have been implanted. Despite the success of VNS to treat drug-resistant epilepsy, the mechanism underlying its effect is incompletely understood.[4]

The vagus nerve is the longest nerve in the human body; it extends from the brainstem to the abdomen. It is composed of 80% afferent fibers and 20% efferent fibers, and aside from the role of the vagus nerve in sensory input and motor control of parts of the pharynx and larynx, it has an important role in the autonomic nervous system. The vagus nerve innervates the heart, lungs, and most if not all of the digestive tract.[5] Most afferent fibers of the vagus nerve are received within the medulla oblongata in the nucleus tractus solitarius (NTS). The NTS in turns projects to the pons, midbrain, and cerebellum as well as the hypothalamic nuclei, thalamic nuclei, amygdala, stria terminalis, and nucleus accumbens of the cerebrum (see **Fig. 1**).[6]

Although the exact mechanism in which VNS therapy reduces seizure activity is not known, significant research has been performed to understand the central effects of the VNS. Multiple experiments have demonstrated that the anticonvulsant effect of the VNS is mediated via the afferent vagal fibers by physically ligating or chemically blocking the efferent vagal fibers distal to the implanted VNS device without alteration in antiseizure function.[7,8] Ascending projections from the vagal nerve may exert central effects on the brainstem structures (NTS, locus coeruleus, and raphe nuclei), and many of these potential mechanisms have all been examined as related to the antiseizure effect.

The NTS is thought to play a central role in VNS mechanism, as among its many projections is the locus coeruleus and the raphae nuclei. Walker and colleagues[9] demonstrated that downregulation of the NTS efferent signal had anticonvulsant effects in a rat model.

Similarly, the role of the locus coeruleus in the VNS mechanism has been examined extensively. Norepinephrine levels are considered to have an antiseizure effect. The locus coeruleus in turn has a regulatory role on central norepinephrine levels.[10] The locus coeruleus was implicated in the mechanism of VNS in an experiment involving the rat model; the anticonvulsant effect of VNS was suppressed when the locus coeruleus was lesioned.[11] Furthermore, VNS was found to increase the discharge rate of the locus coeruleus.[12] VNS has been shown to increase the central concentration of norepinephrine, and increased levels of norepinephrine were associated with therapeutic efficacy.[13]

The central mechanism by which the VNS acts also may be related to effects on the raphe nuclei, which are located in the pons. The raphe nuclei are serotonin-containing cells.[14] Increased serotonin levels have been correlated to decreased seizure activity.[15] Studies have shown that VNS increases the firing rate at the raphe nuclei.[16,17]

Cortical seizures can be induced by applying electrical current to the motor cortex. VNS has been shown to raise the electrical current threshold needed to induce such seizures.[8] Furthermore, low-frequency VNS (below 70 Hz) has been shown to cause desynchronization of the electroencephalograph (EEG) signal.[7] It is hypothesized that the mechanism of action is via pathways from the NTS to the neocortex through structures such as the locus coeruleus.[7]

In addition, the VNS has been shown to alter brain perfusion in multiple studies. PET studies have shown an increase in blood flow to the thalamus and the primary somatosensory cortex and a decrease in blood flow to the limbic system in response to VNS therapy (**Fig. 2**).[18] Functional MRI (fMRI) studies have noted activation in the thalamus, insular cortex, basal ganglia, postcentral gyrus, temporal gyrus, and the inferomedial occipital gyrus with VNS use; the most robust activation has been noted in the thalamus. These studies support the possibility that the VNS mechanism may be related to central changes within the thalamocortical system, which is related to synchronization and propagation of seizure activity.[19]

The timescale in which VNS provides an antiseizure effect sheds light on the central changes it induces. Activation of VNS has been shown to acutely halt seizure activity in less than 5 seconds.[8] When VNS is toggled between stimulation and nonstimulation periods, a therapeutic, antiseizure effect has been demonstrated in the nonstimulation state for periods of up to 10 minutes with corresponding persistent signal changes in the locus coeruleus and blood flow changes in the thalamus.[15,20] On the other hand, VNS has been shown to have increasing anticonvulsant efficacy with long-term use when comparing results at 3 months to 1 year. This increasing antiseizure efficacy has been attributed to a cumulative central effect of VNS therapy.[21] It is likely that multiple mechanisms may contribute to the reduced seizure effect of VNS. On the one hand, VNS causes acute, nearly instantaneous changes in brain function. On the other hand, it leads to long-term central reorganization, both of which appear to decrease seizure activity.

DEPRESSION

After the initial implantation of VNS for treatment of drug-resistant epilepsy, mood changes were observed in recipients unrelated to their response to seizure treatment. In combination with the known antidepressive properties of some antiseizure pharmaceutical agents, Harden and colleagues[22] studied the effect of VNS on mood. As

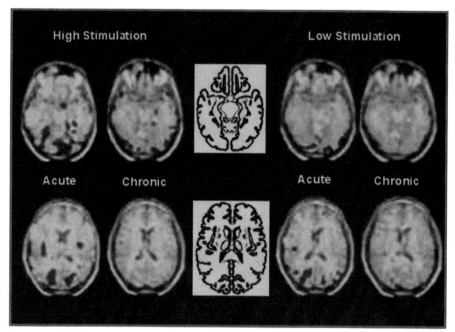

Fig. 2. Cerebral blood flow and VNS. Note that varying stimulation patterns alter cerebral blood flow to specific regions of the brain. This phenomenon may underlie some of the impact that the VNS has had in treating disorders of the CNS. (*From* Henry TR, Bakay RA, Pennell PB, Epstein CM, Votaw JR. Brain blood-flow alterations induced by therapeutic vagus nerve stimulation in partial epilepsy: II. prolonged effects at high and low levels of stimulation. Epilepsia 2004; 45:1064-1070; with permission.)

mentioned previously, VNS alters levels of circulating molecules known to play a role in regulating mood. Thus, it is easy to envision the transition of the VNS as a device for epilepsy to one used to treat depression. Additional studies further evaluated VNS for the treatment of depression, and VNS was ultimately approved as a therapy for chronic and recurrent depression by the FDA in 2005.[4]

It has been postulated that the mechanism by which VNS alters mood in the setting of depression is related to effects on norepinephrine and serotonin levels via the locus coeruleus and raphe nuclei. Brain imaging studies with fMRI and PET have shown varying patterns of changes in activation and blood flow with VNS use. For example, an fMRI study demonstrated activation of the bilateral orbito-frontal and parieto-occipital cortex, the left temporal cortex, the hypothalamus, and the left amygdala.[20] A longitudinal study that examined fludeoxylglucose-18 (FDG) avidity with PET scanning at 3 months and 12 months of VNS therapy for depression demonstrated decreased right-sided dorsolateral prefrontal and cingulate cortical activity followed by increased ventral tegmental area (VTA) activity at 12 months. This may implicate alterations in dopamine levels in the mechanism of VNS for depression as the VTA is the primary brainstem site of dopamine.[23]

OTHER AREAS OF STUDY OF VAGUS NERVE STIMULATION THERAPY

VNS therapy has wide-ranging effects. Due to the wide-ranging effects on the CNS, VNS therapy is being investigated as a possible treatment for a number of other disorders that impact the CNS, including migraine headache, Alzheimer disease, multiple sclerosis, as well as inflammatory-mediated diseases, such as asthma, rheumatoid arthritis, and Crohn disease. Because of animal model findings that support increased neural plasticity with VNS, it is also being examined as a possible treatment for recovery from stroke, posttraumatic stress disorder, and chronic tinnitus.[4,24] The wide range of changes induced by VNS makes the applications of this device almost limitless, and it will be exciting to see what future research will discover next.

CENTRAL EFFECTS OF TRIGEMINAL NERVE STIMULATION

Similar to VNS, trigeminal nerve stimulation (TNS) has shown promising results for treatment of migraine headache, epilepsy, and depression. External TNS (eTNS) has been found effective and has been approved for the treatment of episodic migraine prevention. The TNS mechanism may be similar to that of VNS, as afferent trigeminal nerve fibers are similar to those of the vagus, projecting to the locus coeruleus and the NTS.[7] Compared with healthy volunteers, patients with migraine were found to have hypometabolic functioning in the orbitofrontal (OFC) and rostral anterior cingulate cortices (rACC) on PET imaging. This hypometabolism was reduced after 3 months of use of eTNS in the patients with migraine.[25] rACC activity has been associated with opioid analgesia, and OFC has been implicated in modulation of pain perception.[26,27]

CENTRAL EFFECTS OF COCHLEAR NERVE STIMULATION

Although VNS and TNS are clinically available for their central effects, the most familiar peripheral cranial nerve stimulator to the otolaryngologist is the CI. Although the indications are more clearly defined than with VNS, there are a growing number of subjects worldwide who have benefited from this device. CI was the first-available cranial nerve stimulator, and although time and history have demonstrated that there are undoubtedly central effects that result from CI, these effects are more difficult to measure. MRI and fMRI are not available in human subjects with CI due to image distortion from the magnet. In addition, hearing loss has historically been considered a problem that impacts the peripheral nervous system (eg, spiral ganglion cells, cochlea), and only recently has research begun to explore the impacts on the CNS.[28–30] The field of hearing research seems to be entering an era of transition, whereby research is focusing more on the central impacts of CI that aim to understand how the CNS is processing the sound. In addition, the more global effects of CI are becoming apparent as research is starting to demonstrate associations between hearing loss and cognitive decline.[28–30] This newer research has exciting implications that, much like VNS, broadens the scope of what CI is capable of. Not only does it restore sound input, rather it changes the way sound is perceived and alters central connections that can potentially reverse processes initiated by auditory deprivation. Here we review some of these concepts as we detail the central impact of CI. It is, again, not intended to be comprehensive, rather introductory, as there is an explosion of available research in this area.

COCHLEAR IMPLANTATION

Cochlear implantation provides auditory signal to deafened individuals through direct stimulation of the cochlear nerve. Acoustic signal is encoded via electrical stimulation delivered by a multichannel electrode which is inserted into the cochlea. Stimulation of the electrode bypasses damaged cochlear hair cells to deliver stimulus directly to the cochlear nerve via the spiral ganglion. Multifrequency stimulation is then conveyed from the cochlear nerve to the brainstem, where it travels through the brainstem auditory pathways to the auditory regions of the cortex. Until recently, cochlear implantation precluded use of MRI or magnetoencephalography (MEG). Therefore, the study of central effects of cochlear implantation have been limited compared with VNS. Nevertheless, central changes with CI have been studied with PET, fNIRS (functional near-infrared spectroscopy), EEG, as well as visual and auditory evoked potentials.

After chronic stimulation of the cochlear nerve, cochlear implantees develop central changes that appear consistent with maturation of the central auditory pathways in the cortex and brainstem. Cortical auditory evoked potentials mature in cochlear implantees at a similar rate as those in hearing listeners, when comparing equivalent periods of auditory stimulus.[31] Children with early-onset deafness demonstrate evolution of the auditory brainstem responses after cochlear implantation. After implantation, wave V of the electrically evoked brainstem response was found to mature in a similar fashion as wave V of auditory brainstem response in children with normal hearing.[32]

Central changes have been studied in prelingually and postlingually deafened individuals. fMRI and MEG studies demonstrate that visual cues activate the auditory cortex of prelingually deafened individuals but not of individuals with normal hearing.[33,34] Comparison of cortical activity using PET has shown decreased metabolism in the anterior cingulate gyri, superior temporal cortices, and right parahippocampal gyrus in the postlingually deafened individuals compared with subjects with normal hearing.[35] These cortical changes in the deaf demonstrate cross-modal reorganization: an adaptive reorganization of neural structures to integrate multiple (in this case, visual and auditory) sensory systems (**Fig. 3**).[36] Specifically, there is visual evoked activation of the auditory cortex.

Cross-modal reorganization has been extensively studied in CI recipients. Cochlear implantees have 2 main types of cross-model reorganization. Similar to deaf individuals, there is visual activation of the auditory cortex. Cochlear implantees also have auditory activation of the visual cortex.[37] It is postulated that the auditory activation of the visual cortex may be a beneficial central change, whereas visual takeover of the auditory cortex is a maladaptive plasticity that worsens speech performance in CI users. Studies using PET have demonstrated increased activation of the visual cortex with auditory cues alone in cochlear implantees compared with individuals with normal hearing. The extent of visual cortex activation was correlated with increased time since implantation and with improved speech perception performance.[38] In addition, it has been shown that the "face area" of the visual processing area of the mid-fusiform gyrus is activated in CI listeners in response to auditory speech.[39] A visual evoked potential and EEG study found an inverse relationship between the extent of right auditory cortex activation in response to visual cues and speech performance.[40] Multiple studies using fNIRS and EEG on CI users have found that greater visual cortex reorganization for auditory processing and less auditory cortex changes for visual processing are associated with better speech perception.[41,42]

Comparison of central changes in prelingually and postlingually deafened adult CI recipients may help elucidate reasons for the lack of development of speech comprehension in prelingually deafened adults. A PET study compared cortical activity between prelingually and postlingually deafened adult CI recipients. When listening to speech stimuli, the postlingually deafened adults had increased activation of the left temporal gyrus. In addition, only the postlingually deafened had activation of the Broca area.[43]

Central changes in auditory processing have been studied in children with single-sided deafness (SSD) who have undergone cochlear implantation. EEG

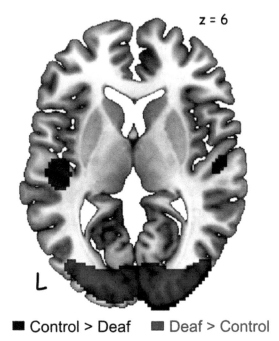

Fig. 3. Adaptation and reorganization of visual and auditory cortices in deafness. In postlingually deafened subjects, the visual cortex is hyperactive and, not surprisingly, the auditory cortex is hypoactive compared with subjects with normal hearing. This reorganization and brain plasticity that occurs demonstrates some of the central changes that occur without hearing. (*From* Han JH, Lee HJ, Kang H, Oh SH, Lee DS .Brain Plasticity can Predict the Cochlear Implant Outcome in Adult-Onset Deafness. Front Hum Neurosci. 2019 Feb 19;13:38; with permission.)

measurements of SSD children demonstrated preferential activity of a unilateral auditory cortex immediately following cochlear implantation. With chronic stimulation, the children demonstrated contralateral aural preference in each auditory cortex.[44] Early SSD CI may improve binaural hearing by promoting bilateral auditory cortex utilization.

DISCUSSION

Stimulation of the vagus nerve has clinically important therapeutic effects on epilepsy and depression. Although the mechanism of action of VNS is not fully understood, there appear to be significant central changes throughout the brain, including the brainstem and areas of the cortex. Further elucidating the central changes caused by VNS may allow for improved efficacy of VNS therapy for epilepsy and depression as well as expanded indications for VNS.

Cochlear nerve stimulation via the CI restores sound perception to deafened individuals. The ability to understand speech with cochlear implantation is related to patient-specific characteristics (eg, prelingual or postlingual deafness, duration of deafness, age) as well as reorganization of central auditory pathways. Further research on the central effects of cochlear implantation may help predict those who will most benefit from cochlear implantation and may inform aural rehabilitation programs that aim to maximize reorganization of central auditory pathways to achieve better speech perception.

Based on substantial, evolving evidence, from vagus and cochlear nerve stimulators, cranial nerve stimulation appears to cause wide, sometimes unexpected central changes. Some of these central changes have led to additional therapeutics; for example, VNS to treat depression and headache. The central effects of newer cranial nerve stimulators, such as hypoglossal, recurrent laryngeal, and vestibular, will need to be studied, as these newer peripheral nerve stimulators reach the clinical setting. The effects of cranial nerve stimulators may, indeed, be much broader than the initial clinical targets. The potential conditions that could benefit from central effects of peripheral cranial nerve stimulation is vast and the prospect of discovering further positive impacts from these stimulators makes the future bright.

REFERENCES

1. Guinand N, van de Berg R, Cavuscens S, et al. Vestibular implants: 8 years of experience with electrical stimulation of the vestibular nerve in 11 patients with bilateral vestibular loss. ORL J Otorhinolaryngol Relat Spec 2015;77:227–40.
2. Svensson P, Romaniello A, Wang K, et al. One hour of tongue-task training is associated with plasticity in corticomotor control of the human tongue musculature. Exp Brain Res 2006;173:165–73.
3. Zanchetti A, Wang SC, Moruzzi G. The effect of vagal afferent stimulation on the EEG pattern of the cat. Electroencephalogr Clin Neurophysiol 1952;4:357–61.
4. Johnson RL, Wilson CG. A review of vagus nerve stimulation as a therapeutic intervention. J Inflamm Res 2018;11:203–13.
5. Bonaz B, Sinniger V, Pellissier S. Anti-inflammatory properties of the vagus nerve: potential therapeutic implications of vagus nerve stimulation. J Physiol 2016;594: 5781–90.
6. Henry TR. Therapeutic mechanisms of vagus nerve stimulation. Neurology 2002; 59:S3–14.
7. Fanselow EE. Central mechanisms of cranial nerve stimulation for epilepsy. Surg Neurol Int 2012;3:S247–54.
8. Zabara J. Inhibition of experimental seizures in canines by repetitive vagal stimulation. Epilepsia 1992;33:1005–12.
9. Walker BR, Easton A, Gale K. Regulation of limbic motor seizures by GABA and glutamate transmission in nucleus tractus solitarius. Epilepsia 1999;40:1051–7.
10. Fornai F, Ruffoli R, Giorgi FS, et al. The role of locus coeruleus in the antiepileptic activity induced by vagus nerve stimulation. Eur J Neurosci 2011;33:2169–78.
11. Krahl SE, Clark KB, Smith DC, et al. Locus coeruleus lesions suppress the seizure-attenuating effects of vagus nerve stimulation. Epilepsia 1998;39:709–14.
12. Groves DA, Bowman EM, Brown VJ. Recordings from the rat locus coeruleus during acute vagal nerve stimulation in the anaesthetised rat. Neurosci Lett 2005; 379:174–9.
13. Raedt R, Clinckers R, Mollet L, et al. Increased hippocampal noradrenaline is a biomarker for efficacy of vagus nerve stimulation in a limbic seizure model. J Neurochem 2011;117:461–9.
14. Hornung JP. The human raphe nuclei and the serotonergic system. J Chem Neuroanat 2003;26:331–43.
15. Bagdy G, Kecskemeti V, Riba P, et al. Serotonin and epilepsy. J Neurochem 2007; 100:857–73.
16. Dorr AE, Debonnel G. Effect of vagus nerve stimulation on serotonergic and noradrenergic transmission. J Pharmacol Exp Ther 2006;318:890–8.

17. Manta S, El Mansari M, Blier P. Novel attempts to optimize vagus nerve stimulation parameters on serotonin neuronal firing activity in the rat brain. Brain Stimul 2012;5:422–9.

18. Henry TR, Bakay RA, Pennell PB, et al. Brain blood-flow alterations induced by therapeutic vagus nerve stimulation in partial epilepsy: II. prolonged effects at high and low levels of stimulation. Epilepsia 2004;45:1064–70.

19. Narayanan JT, Watts R, Haddad N, et al. Cerebral activation during vagus nerve stimulation: a functional MR study. Epilepsia 2002;43:1509–14.

20. Bohning DE, Lomarev MP, Denslow S, et al. Feasibility of vagus nerve stimulation-synchronized blood oxygenation level-dependent functional MRI. Invest Radiol 2001;36:470–9.

21. DeGiorgio CM, Schachter SC, Handforth A, et al. Prospective long-term study of vagus nerve stimulation for the treatment of refractory seizures. Epilepsia 2000; 41:1195–200.

22. Harden CL, Pulver MC, Ravdin LD, et al. A pilot study of mood in epilepsy patients treated with vagus nerve stimulation. Epilepsy Behav 2000;1:93–9.

23. Conway CR, Chibnall JT, Gebara MA, et al. Association of cerebral metabolic activity changes with vagus nerve stimulation antidepressant response in treatment-resistant depression. Brain Stimul 2013;6:788–97.

24. Hays SA, Rennaker RL, Kilgard MP. Targeting plasticity with vagus nerve stimulation to treat neurological disease. Prog Brain Res 2013;207:275–99.

25. Magis D, D'Ostilio K, Thibaut A, et al. Cerebral metabolism before and after external trigeminal nerve stimulation in episodic migraine. Cephalalgia 2017;37: 881–91.

26. Becker S, Gandhi W, Pomares F, et al. Orbitofrontal cortex mediates pain inhibition by monetary reward. Soc Cogn Affect Neurosci 2017;12:651–61.

27. Petrovic P, Kalso E, Petersson KM, et al. Placebo and opioid analgesia–imaging a shared neuronal network. Science 2002;295:1737–40.

28. Armstrong NM, An Y, Ferrucci L, et al. Temporal sequence of hearing impairment and cognition in the Baltimore longitudinal study of aging. J Gerontol A Biol Sci Med Sci 2018. [Epub ahead of print].

29. Brenowitz WD, Kaup AR, Lin FR, et al. Multiple sensory impairment is associated with increased risk of dementia among black and white older adults. J Gerontol A Biol Sci Med Sci 2019;74:890–6.

30. Deal JA, Goman AM, Albert MS, et al. Hearing treatment for reducing cognitive decline: design and methods of the aging and cognitive health evaluation in elders randomized controlled trial. Alzheimers Dement (N Y) 2018;4:499–507.

31. Ponton CW, Eggermont JJ. Of kittens and kids: altered cortical maturation following profound deafness and cochlear implant use. Audiol Neurootol 2001; 6:363–80.

32. Thai-Van H, Cozma S, Boutitie F, et al. The pattern of auditory brainstem response wave V maturation in cochlear-implanted children. Clin Neurophysiol 2007;118: 676–89.

33. Finney EM, Clementz BA, Hickok G, et al. Visual stimuli activate auditory cortex in deaf subjects: evidence from MEG. Neuroreport 2003;14:1425–7.

34. Finney EM, Fine I, Dobkins KR. Visual stimuli activate auditory cortex in the deaf. Nat Neurosci 2001;4:1171–3.

35. Lee JS, Lee DS, Oh SH, et al. PET evidence of neuroplasticity in adult auditory cortex of postlingual deafness. J Nucl Med 2003;44:1435–9.

36. Han JH, Lee HJ, Kang H, et al. Brain plasticity can predict the cochlear implant outcome in adult-onset deafness. Front Hum Neurosci 2019;13:38.

37. Campbell J, Sharma A. Visual cross-modal re-organization in children with cochlear implants. PLoS One 2016;11:e0147793.
38. Giraud AL, Price CJ, Graham JM, et al. Cross-modal plasticity underpins language recovery after cochlear implantation. Neuron 2001;30:657–63.
39. Giraud AL, Truy E. The contribution of visual areas to speech comprehension: a PET study in cochlear implants patients and normal-hearing subjects. Neuropsychologia 2002;40:1562–9.
40. Sandmann P, Dillier N, Eichele T, et al. Visual activation of auditory cortex reflects maladaptive plasticity in cochlear implant users. Brain 2012;135:555–68.
41. Chen LC, Puschmann S, Debener S. Increased cross-modal functional connectivity in cochlear implant users. Sci Rep 2017;7:10043.
42. Chen LC, Sandmann P, Thorne JD, et al. Cross-modal functional reorganization of visual and auditory cortex in adult cochlear implant users identified with fNIRS. Neural Plast 2016;2016:4382656.
43. Petersen B, Gjedde A, Wallentin M, et al. Cortical plasticity after cochlear implantation. Neural Plast 2013;2013:318521.
44. Polonenko MJ, Gordon KA, Cushing SL, et al. Cortical organization restored by cochlear implantation in young children with single sided deafness. Sci Rep 2017;7:16900.

Special Considerations in Patients with Cranial Neurostimulatory Implants

Johanna L. Wickemeyer, MD[a], Jeffrey D. Sharon, MD[b],
Heather M. Weinreich, MD, MPH[a],*

KEYWORDS

- Cochlear implant • MRI • Safety • Image quality • Interaction
- Auditory brainstem implant • Magnet

KEY POINTS

- MRI magnets can interfere with cochlear implants, causing imaging artifacts, pain, and device complications.
- Cochlear implants can interfere with other devices, such as ventriculoperitoneal shunts.
- Newer neurostimulatory devices, such as the hypoglossal nerve stimulator and vagal stimulator, require further study for potential interactions.

INTRODUCTION

In this article, we explore the special considerations related to implantable devices in the head and neck, including cochlear implants (CIs), auditory brainstem implants (ABIs), and stimulators of hypoglossal, vagal, vestibular, and olfactory nerves. One of the most significant considerations pertains to MRI use with these implants. MRIs use radiofrequency pulses to excite hydrogen nuclei within a powerful magnetic field. Implants with ferromagnetic metals or an implanted magnet can interact with this field risking projectile effects, twisting of the device, heating, image artifacts, demagnetization, and device malfunctions.[1,2]

COCHLEAR IMPLANTS

- At the time of writing, each CI manufacturer has an MR Conditional device that is approved for 1.5-T or 3.0-T scans with the magnet in place

Disclosures: Authors do not have any disclosures or funding to report regarding the preparation of this article.
[a] Department of Otolaryngology–Head and Neck Surgery, University of Illinois – Chicago, 1855 West Taylor Street, MC 648, Chicago, IL 60612, USA; [b] Department of Otolaryngology–Head and Neck Surgery, University of California San Francisco, 2233 Post Street, San Francisco, CA 94115, USA
* Corresponding author.
E-mail address: hweinre1@uic.edu

Otolaryngol Clin N Am 53 (2020) 57–71
https://doi.org/10.1016/j.otc.2019.09.013
0030-6665/20/© 2019 Elsevier Inc. All rights reserved.

- Older-generation CIs are not as MR compatible, and familiarity with manufacturer's recommendations for each device is recommended
- CIs create MRI artifacts, and certain imaging strategies can help maximize image quality

CIs are used in management of sensorineural hearing loss by bypassing the cochlea to electrically stimulate the cochlear nerve. From the time the first implant was placed by Dr William House in 1961[3] to 2019, more than 324,000 CIs have been implanted.[4] It is widely considered to be the most successful neural implant in the world. However, because of the need for precise alignment of the outer and inner coils, the internal and external device each contain a magnet. This can result in interaction with other devices with magnets, such as MRI and programmable shunts.

Imaging

The chance of a CI recipient requiring an MRI scan in his or her lifetime is estimated to be between 50% and 75%.[5] In the past, surgical magnet removal from the internal device before scanning was standard for many devices, although for devices without a removable magnet, MR was contraindicated. However, magnet removal carried risk of infection and delayed device use while the incision healed.[1] Initial testing of force, heating, and quality of imaging[6] were first studied in the 1990s with demonstration of limited safety of CIs in scanners. Early studies were mixed, with some advising against MRIs due to internal device movement,[7] whereas others[8] demonstrated minimal movement and overall safety at 1.5 T.

The Food and Drug Administration (FDA) MRI safety labeling has 3 categories. MR Unsafe denotes that devices are unsafe and should not be scanned. MR Conditional indicates approval for MR under very specific circumstances that need to be followed. MR Safe denotes that the device should not interact with MR and that there are no restrictions or safety concerns. In 2013, the FDA approved the MED-EL (Innsbruck, Austria) Concert, Pulsar, and Sonata as MR Conditional at 1.5 T. In 2015, the MED-EL Synchrony was approved as MR Conditional at 3T without requiring magnet removal or head splint wrap.[9] This was possible because of a new magnet design, whereby the internal magnet could spin within its housing to self-align within the magnetic field of the scanner (**Fig. 1**). With enhanced alignment of the magnet within the magnetic field, forces acting on the internal device

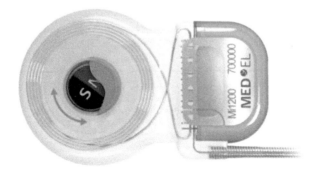

Fig. 1. Design of the MED-EL magnet. The polarity of the magnet allows for rotation with the magnetic field (noted by *arrow*). (*Courtesy of* MED-EL, Innsbruck, Austria; with permission.)

are minimized. In 2018, the Advanced Bionics (Valencia, CA) HiRes Ultra 3D was FDA approved for 3T MRI. The design of this magnet array allows for each magnet to freely rotate, resulting in decreased device torque (**Fig. 2**). In 2019, Cochlear (Sydney, Australia) received FDA approval for the 3T MRI compatible Profile Plus implant series.

All 3 manufacturers (Advanced Bionics, Cochlear, and MED-EL) provide MRI compatibility instructions for each device (**Table 1**). All manufacturers advise MRI to be performed at least 6 months after initial surgical implantation.

It is critical the surgeon and radiology team be familiar with the specific implant and review the company's published device specifications before allowing any CI patient in an MRI scanner. The patient and the ordering clinician (if not the implant surgeon) should be counseled on risks and benefits of undergoing MRI with the implants in place. Usage of alternate imaging modalities, like ultrasound or computed tomography, should be considered if they will provide equivalent diagnostic information. Potential risks of CI use in MRIs include the following: device movement with possible extrusion, pain, discomfort over site, poor quality of imaging, device malfunction, demagnetization, wound or skin changes. Open communication between patient, otolaryngologist, and radiologist is very helpful. If the patient agrees to undergo a scan with a magnet in place against the manufacturer's recommendation, then the patient should be made aware of that, and informed consent and proper documentation are recommended. If the identity of the internal device is not clear from the patient or records, then a plain film of the skull can often clarify some basic information, as each device has recognizable markings. In addition, the authors have found it helpful to create an imaging protocol with their radiologists.

Safety

MRI use and safety are still being evaluated. The literature is composed of retrospective case series with one prospective study.[10] Most images involve 1.5-T MRI. Published complication rates are low.[1,6–8,10–15] Magnet displacement is the most common concern.[1,13] A Japanese study demonstrated the measured displacement force and torque on the Pulsar and Concerto magnets were less than values reported in the CI manual.[16] In a study of 19 ears in 34 MRI scans, internal magnet movement, "flipping" occurred in up to 15% of cases.[13] Other adverse events include return to the operating room for magnet removal and intolerable pain. In studies, the Synchrony with its rotating and self-aligning magnet (see **Fig. 1**), had fewer complications as compared with the older (nonrotating) magnet designs.[1]

Pain

Up to 70% of patients with a CI experience pain during an MRI scan.[10,15] Pain can occur while moving in or out of the scanner, as well as during image acquisition.[10]

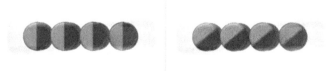

Fig. 2. Array of freely rotating magnet schema in Advanced Bionics HiRes Ultra 3D. (*Courtesy of* Advanced Bionics AG and affiliates, California; with permission.)

Table 1
MRI compatibility of cochlear implant devices approved by the food and drug administration

Manufacturer	CI Model	Tesla	
		1.5 T	3.0 T
Cochlear Nucleus*	Profile Plus	Yes, magnet in place without headwrap	Yes, magnet in place without headwrap
	Profile	Yes, magnet in place with headwrap/MR Kit	Yes, with removal of magnet
	Freedom	Yes, magnet in place with headwrap/MR Kit	Yes, with removal of magnet
Advanced Bionics^	HiRes Ultra 3D	Yes, magnet in place without headwrap	Yes, magnet in place without headwrap
	HiRes Ultra	Yes, magnet in place without headwrap	Yes, with removal of magnet
	HiRes 90K	Yes, with removal of magnet	Yes, with removal of magnet
MED-EL+	Synchrony	Yes, magnet in place without headwrap	Yes, magnet in place without headwrap
	Concerto	Yes, magnet in place with headwrap	No
	Sonata	Yes, magnet in place with headwrap	No

Note that information is accurate at the time of writing in August 2019.

* Information in chart pertaining to that manufacturer obtained from: https://www.cochlear.com/intl/home.

^ Information in chart pertaining to that manufacturer obtained from: https://www.cochlear.com/intl/home.

+ Information in chart pertaining to that manufacturer obtained from: https://www.medel.com/us/.

Pain, due to the magnet pull within the field, can occur regardless of the image's anatomic location (eg, brain, lower extremity).[10,15] Pain can also be secondary to the tightness of the headwrap.[10,15]

Pain has been described as "pressure," "heat," or "sharp," and is typically less than 5 on a 10-point scale. Most patients can tolerate the MRI without sedation[10,11,13,14] and even without a headwrap.[17,18] Several CI magnet types, such as the diametrically bipolar magnet in the Synchrony result in little to no reported pain.

An estimated at 88% of MRI scans can be completed even in the setting of pain.[10] Most patients prefer this than undergoing surgical magnet removal.[10] All patients should be properly counseled on the risk of pain while in the MRI. Some clinicians advise the use of an over-the-counter analgesic for patient comfort. Injection of local anesthetics may relieve pain; however, this may mask pain, which may be the only indicator of trauma to surrounding tissue or issues with the magnet.

In published studies examining efficacy and safety of device wrapping, most CIs included were not approved for MRI, and device wrapping was considered "off label." In studies, the wrapping material varied. In the authors' practice, for older-generation CIs, a head wrap consisted of a firm "puck" of hearing aid model material followed by placement of 3M (Maplewood, MN) Ioban 2 Antimicrobial Incise Drape around the head and secured with 3M Micropore Surgical Tape (**Fig. 3**). For many MR Conditional devices, the manufacturer will provide a kit with a headwrap if indicated.

For any device, regardless of generation, a clinician should be available while the patient is undergoing the scan and should evaluate the patient's pain and implant

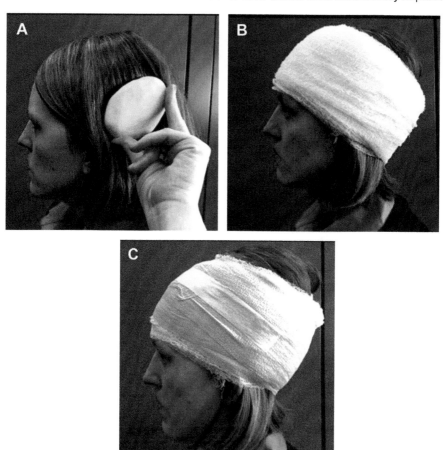

Fig. 3. Noncompany headwrap for CI is shown. (*A*) First, the silicone rubber mold is custom made for each patient. (*B*) Next, the head is wrapped with woven gauze. (*C*) The head wrapped in the gauze.

site afterward. The external processor should be placed to determine the magnet polarity and functionality of the device. If there are any concerns, imaging is warranted. A plain film of the skull is generally sufficient to see a magnet displacement (**Fig. 4**). Movement of the magnet may be addressed by manipulation of magnet, reducing it back into place. If this is not able to be performed, surgical correction is required.

Image quality
Image quality can be compromised due to the internal magnet or metal artifact. Even with magnet removal, the internal receiver causes artifact (**Fig. 5**). Conditions such as stroke, tumors, and structural abnormalities may warrant routine surveillance scans and quality of imaging may be not useful. The potential for artifact needs to be included in preoperative discussions.[17]

Sharon and colleagues[19] examined MRI quality with CIs in 57 MRI brain images with 765 sequences. Reviewed images were graded as to the view of the ipsilateral and contralateral internal auditory canal (IAC) and whether or not the scan was felt to be of sufficient quality to answer the question for which it was ordered. For viewing

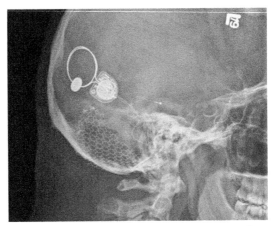

Fig. 4. Displaced magnet is visible on plain film after MR scan. Titanium cranioplasty is also visible.

ipsilateral IAC and cerebellopontine angle (CPA), scans that (1) acquired multiple planes of imaging, (2) had high-resolution images, and (3) acquired multiple sequences had the highest odds of producing useable images. In addition, fat saturation algorithms seemed to produce a secondary artifact that significantly degraded image quality (**Fig. 6**). Diffusion-weighted imaging (DWI) was highly susceptible to magnet artifact and were generally unusable (**Fig. 7**). This is important when considering the indication for the scan, as stroke and cholesteatoma detection can rely on DWI. Overall, high-resolution, post-contrast coronal image sequences had the highest odds of producing suitable images of the ipsilateral IAC and CPA for tumor detection. Other studies[1] have corroborated these findings, showing multiple sequences, high-resolution sequences, multiple planes of acquisition, and avoiding DWIs as the most useful options for optimizing image quality. They also found that artifact with heavily T2-weighted sequences varied by manufacturer. As devices become increasingly compatible for MR scans with the internal magnet in situ, more work will be needed to optimize imaging parameters and algorithms for this

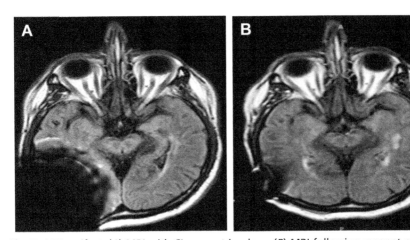

Fig. 5. MRI artifact. (*A*) MRI with CI magnet in place. (*B*) MRI following magnet removal.

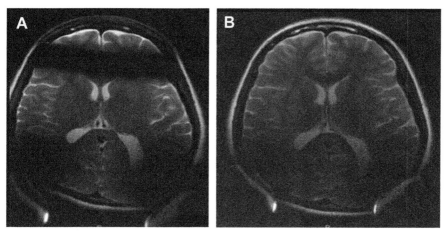

Fig. 6. Fat saturation algorithms. (*A*) Fat saturation algorithm causing artifact. (*B*) Same sequence without fat saturation algorithm.

unique patient population. If a high-quality scan is required, magnet removal remains an option.

Radiation

X-ray
Doses used in medical imaging are not considered to be high enough energy to directly damage the implant.

Radiotherapy
Radiotherapy, a form of ionizing radiation, uses mainly gamma rays, which are shorter in wavelength to common x-rays. Gamma rays can destroy the atomic grid of semi-conductors in the CI. Doses of up to 50 Gy do not cause damage to the implant or change total current output.[20,21] Depending on the manufacturer, CIs can withstand between 240 and 250 Gy using 6 to 15 MV photon beam strength.[22,23] Direct contact

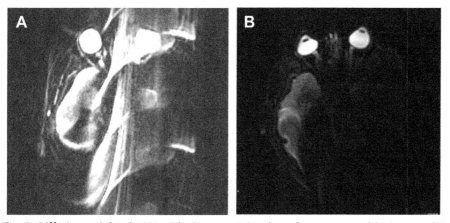

Fig. 7. Diffusion-weighted MRI with CI magnet in place show non-useable images. (*A*) Apparent diffusion coefficient map. (*B*) Diffusion-weighted image.

of the beam with the device may concentrate the energy, resulting in tissue necrosis.[22,23] In general, the radiation beam should avoid the implant as much as possible.

Proton therapy
Photons, created in a cyclotron, are directed to tumor cells by magnetic fields that may interact with the CI.[24] Similar to gamma rays, proton beams can destroy the atomic grid of semiconductors in CI, and therefore CI should not be in the direct pathway of the beam if possible.

Radioisotope therapy
Radioisotope therapy uses the natural decay process of the radioactive material to emit radioactive rays. Commonly used in head and neck cancer is Iodine-131 for the treatment of thyroid cancer. The use of this therapy poses a theoretic risk to the CI. Radioisotope therapy is similar to gamma rays and proton beams, and radioisotopes have the potential to destroy the atomic grid of semiconductors in a CI.

Functional scintigraphy
Functional scintigraphy uses radioactive isotopes as a tracer. The tracer, taken up by tissue undergoing rapid change, emits low levels of gamma rays. These gamma rays are low energy and are safe to be used in CI recipients.

Ultrasound
Diagnostic ultrasound may be safely used in the patient with a CI. However, ultrasound therapy and imaging should not be used directly in the area of the implant, as the device can theoretically concentrate the ultrasound field causing damage to surrounding tissue. Depending on the manufacturer, the parameters of energy can be between 500 and 15,000 W/m^2 and within a frequency of 2 to 5 MHz.[22,23]

Occupational
Occupational exposure to ionizing radiation is regulated, as continuous exposure may accumulate in the body. This exposure should be monitored and should not preclude CI recipients from these positions.

Implantable Devices
Possible interactions may occur, and a patient undergoing a CI or who is receiving another implant, needs to be counseled. These are summarized in **Table 2**.

Valve shunt
Valve shunt systems are used to relieve cerebrospinal fluid (CSF) pressure in hydrocephalus. Some shunt systems are controlled by a programmable valve that is managed by an external device with a magnetic link. The CI magnet has the capability to interact with the valve setting.[24] This dangerous interaction has been demonstrated in both human and cadaveric studies.[22–24] In July 2019, the FDA released a statement regarding this potential interaction, warning that inadvertent changes in the settings of the pump by the CI may result in under-drainage or over-drainage of CSF.[25] The CI and shunt device must be evaluated in conjunction, and manufacturer specifications must be reviewed to determine safety. Recipients and potential recipients should be made aware of this interaction. Valve settings on the shunt should be checked and monitored on a scheduled basis. The FDA advises placing the shunt on the contralateral side of the CI, or, in the case of bilateral CIs, placing it a maximum distance from the ipsilateral CI. Studies suggest that implantation may be safely performed if the devices are placed more than 1 cm apart.[26,27]

Table 2
Co-implant interactions with cochlear implants (CIs)

Device	Background	Theoretic Interaction	Reports	Recommendations
Valve shunt system (VSS)	Programmable VSS use magnetic switches to control drainage rate	CI coil has the capability to interact with the valve setting	Demonstrated interaction[26,27]	Food and Drug Administration recommends: • Educate patients • Scheduled shunt valve settings • Placement of shunt relative to CI
Implantable drug pump	Pumps uses radiofrequency signals for programming	CI programming could interact with pump programming and vice versa	None	Special care should be taken with programming of each device to avoid interference
Pacemaker/implantable cardioverter-defibrillator (ICD)	Some pacemakers and ICDs have magnetically activated switch	Programmable switch on pacemakers/ICD may be impacted by the presence of magnet	No interference[28,29]	CI magnets and/or remote magnets should be at least 15 cm from pacemaker/ICD
Implantable pulse generator (IPG)	IPGs use implanted electrodes	Conduction of current between IPG and CI	None	IPG electrodes should be place >1 cm away from CI
Deep brain stimulator (DBS)	DBS function from a localized, bipolar stimulation and may use a magnetic switch	DBS may use a magnetic switch which could be impacted by the CI magnet	No interference[30]	Consult the DBS manufacturer
Vagus nerve stimulator	Stimulus output is controlled with magnetic switch	CI could disinhibited switch, causing constitutive vagal nerve stimulation	None	CI magnets >15 cm away from the vagal nerve stimulator
Vascular clips, bone screws/plates, heart valves	Common intraoperative implants are made of metallic alloys (ie, titanium, cobalt, stainless steel)	Diamagnetic implants could result in magnetic attraction of cochlear implant	None	No interaction is expected and can be used CI recipients
Traditional hearing aid (HA), bone-conductive hearing aid	Some HAs use inductive transmission technology through telecoil for programming	CI radiofrequency may interfere with transmission, preventing control or programming	None	Alter position of HA or hand-held device

Implantable drug pumps

Implantable drug pumps are used to administer intrathecal medication. Pumps typically use radiofrequency signals for programming. The radiofrequency of the CI has the potential to interact with that of the pump, and vice versa.[24] Special care should be taken with programming of each device to avoid interference.

Cardiac pacemakers/implantable cardioverter-defibrillator

In some pacemakers and implantable cardioverter-defibrillators (ICDs), the programming switch is magnetically activated. The CI's sound processor coil or remote could interact with the pacemaker switch. Unipolar-sensing or single lead pacemakers and ICDs are more prone to electromagnetic interference. Theoretically, CIs operating at a low stimulation rate could impact the programming of a unipolar pacemaker electrode. From the minimal research that exists, CIs can be safely placed in patients with cardiac pacemakers.[28,29] It is advised that pacemaker coils and remote assistant wands be placed at least 15 cm away from the CI magnet to decrease electromagnetic interference.[24]

Implantable pulse generator

Implantable pulse generators (IPGs) have implanted electrodes that stimulate and target specific areas of the body. The electrode used is typically a bipolar stimulation. CIs may impact the function of the pulse generator. Similar to electrocautery, the current conducted between the IPG and the implant could damage the CI or surrounding tissue. The electrode of the IPG should not be placed directly on the implant and should be at least 1 cm away from the implant.

Deep brain stimulator

Deep brain stimulators (DBSs), used in the treatment of Parkinson disease, may use a battery-operated localized bipolar stimulator. The distance from the stimulated area within the brain is usually at a sufficient distance from the CI site (**Fig. 8**). DBSs have been found to have no interaction with CIs, as the CI magnet is not of sufficient strength to affect the magnetic lead switch within the DBS.[24,30] The DBS manufacturer should be consulted on the effect of the CI implant on the stimulator.

Vagus nerve stimulator

The vagus nerve stimulator (VNS) delivers a current that is not impacted by a CI. The stimulus output of the stimulator is controlled with a magnetic switch and theoretically the CI magnet could interfere. It the switch is disinhibited, the stimulator can fire constantly, resulting in vagal nerve deterioration. The CI magnet should be kept a minimum of 15 cm away from the stimulator.

Vascular clips, bone screws/plates, heart valves

Many intraoperative implants are made of metallic alloys. Diamagnetic implants could result in magnetic attraction of the CI; however, inference and magnetic attraction have not been described in the literature.

Traditional hearing aid, bone-conductive hearing aid

CI recipients may continue to wear a conventional hearing aid in the contralateral ear. The aids may use inductive transmission technology through a telecoil for programming. The radiofrequency produced by the CI may interfere with transmission. An audiologist may alter position of these devices so that the hearing aid can be properly controlled or programmed. There are no interactions expected from a bone-conduction or implantable hearing aids.

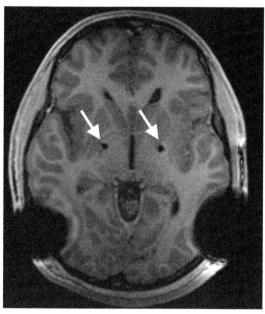

Fig. 8. MRI of a 17-year-old male patient with a congenital condition that resulted in dystonia and deafness. The patient underwent bilateral cochlear implantation before DBS placement for treatment of dystonia. MRI demonstrates CI artifact after removal of magnets, as well as bilateral DBS leads are visible in the globus pallidi/basal ganglia (denoted by *white arrows*).

Other Interactions with Cochlear Implants

Cautery

Electrosurgical instruments can produce high-frequency voltages and direct coupling might occur between the cautery tip and the CI electrode. The currents produced by cautery have the capability to damage the implant or surrounding tissues. CI manufacturers recommend avoiding monopolar cautery in the head and neck; however, there are no published case reports of CI dysfunction. Bipolar may be used if the probe tips are kept more than 1 to 5 mm away from the implant.[22,23]

Airport security

CIs may set off standard airport metal detectors. Newer tools, such as millimeter wave scanners, use electromagnetic radiation, whereas backscatter x-rays use ionizing radiation. The radiation amount emitted is low and will not damage the implant. The electromagnetic fields produced by these tools may interact with microphone input to the sound processor, resulting in distorted sound. During screening, the device can be turned off to avoid distortion and all patients should carry their device identification card with them.

Electrotherapies

Electroshock or convulsive therapies, used to treat depression, mania, and catatonia, are contraindicated in CI recipients, as they may damage the implant or the cochlea. Electrical stimulation instruments, such as neurostimulation and transcutaneous electrical nerve/muscle stimulation, should not be directly placed over the implant. If the device uses bipolar stimulation, it may be used within 1 cm of the CI.[22–24]

AUDITORY BRAINSTEM IMPLANTS

ABIs directly stimulate the cochlear nucleus and are indicated for patients with an absent cochlear nerve. The Nucleus ABI for patients with Neurofibromatosis type 2 (NF2) is the only FDA-approved device. Given the multitude of intracranial tumors with NF2, MRI is critical in managing these patients. Like CIs, ABIs contain an implantable receiver with magnet that can impact safety and image quality. For MRIs, the nucleus requires surgical removal of the internal magnet or external compression to minimize magnet displacement.

Data on MRI safety with ABIs are limited because of low numbers of implantees. Findings are similar to the CI literature and most patients undergo imaging without any adverse events. Some patients experience pain or movement of the magnet, requiring local anesthesia or surgical removal of the magnet.[1,12,31] The imaging artifact generally affects only the ipsilateral view. In certain sequences, such as axial 3-dimensional inversion recovery prepared fast spoiled gradient echo, coronal T1, and axial T1, the ipsilateral cerebellopontine angles and IAC are well-visualized in 85% of cases. Sequences other than the ones listed showed only the ipsilateral IAC-CPA in fewer than 50% of cases studied.[12]

HYPOGLOSSAL NERVE STIMULATOR

The hypoglossal nerve stimulator is used in the treatment of obstructive sleep apnea. There are 3 types of hypoglossal nerve stimulator system, only one of which was FDA approved in 2014. The Inspire II Upper Airway Stimulation device (Inspire Medical Systems, Inc., Maple Grove, MN) consists of a stimulation lead attached to the distal hypoglossal nerve, an intercostal sensing lead to detect the respiratory cycle, and a pulse generator on the anterior chest wall inferior to the clavicle.[32]

The Inspire Model 3028 generator system is MR Conditional in a 1.5-T MRI, with the following restrictions. MRI should include only head or extremities and should not include the device. There are specific requirements in terms of the coils used and the manufacturer's guide should be referenced. The Model 3024 is MR Unsafe.[33]

Potential MRI imaging complications include the following: lead electrode or generator heating resulting in tissue damage, induced currents on leads, damage to the generator or leads causing failure or overstimulation of the system, and movement or vibration of the generator or leads.

As hypoglossal nerve stimulation is an emerging entity and candidacy remains strict, little is known of comorbidities and co-implantation. A small case series demonstrated dysfunction of the hypoglossal nerve stimulator with electrocardioversion for atrial fibrillation[34]; however, one patient with electroconvulsive therapy for bipolar depression saw no change in device functionality.[35]

VAGAL NERVE STIMULATORS

VNSs are used in the treatment of medication-resistant epilepsy and depression and stimulate the nerve via implanted or transcutaneous device. For an implanted VNS, an electrode, wrapped around the vagal nerve, is attached to a pulse generator. For a transcutaneous VNS, the auricular branch of the vagus nerve is stimulated via the external auditory meatus and cymba/cavum conchae. The Cyberonics (Houston, TX) VNS is the only currently approved device.[36]

Due to the history of epilepsy, MRIs are routinely indicated in this population. The Cyberonics VNS is MR Conditional 1.5-T and 3.0-T MRI with a head-only transmit coil. To prevent undesired stimulation during the scan, the VNS must be programmed to magnet mode output of 0 mA.[36,37] Although patients may not experience complications,[37] image quality may be compromised. MRI scans of 3 T requiring head coil and protocols including 3-dimensional fluid-attenuated inversion recovery took longer with loss of the contrast effectiveness leading to poor quality.[38]

OTHER NEURAL STIMULATORS
Vestibular Implant

The vestibular implant translates rotational acceleration into an electrical stimulus that is transferred to the 3 ampullary nerves, with the goal of treating bilateral loss of vestibular function. Trials involving vestibular implants are ongoing at the time of writing; they are not yet FDA approved. The recently developed Multichannel Vestibular Implant (provided by Labyrinth Device, LLC) is based on the Concerto and includes a Concerto magnet and 2 VORP magnets (which are the same magnets used in the MED-EL VIBRANT SOUNDBRIDGE). Although the MED-EL Concerto, MED-EL VIBRANT SOUNDBRIDGE, and Cochlear Nucleus Freedom are considered MRI conditional in the United States, the designation requires testing that has not yet been performed with the specific implant devices at this time of this writing.[39]

Olfactory Nerve Stimulator

Electrical stimulation of the olfactory bulb is still in development, and given the exploratory nature of the device, no known special considerations are considered.[40]

SUMMARY

As more individuals receive neural implants including CIs, clinicians need to be aware of safety risks these devices pose. From metallic materials to magnets, these devices can alter imaging, interfere with other devices, and put patients at risk. To ensure patient safety, clinicians need to be familiar with each device and should review manufacturer guidelines before implanting. Known potential interactions and safety concerns should be discussed with the patient before implantation of a new device.

REFERENCES

1. Shew M, Wichova H, Lin J, et al. Magnetic resonance imaging with cochlear implants and auditory brainstem implants: are we truly practicing MRI safety? Laryngoscope 2019;129(2):482–9.
2. Tang Q, Li Y. MRI compatibility and safety of cochlear implants. Zhong Nan Da Xue Xue Bao Yi Xue Ban 2012;37(3):311–5.
3. Eshraghi AA, Nazarian R, Telischi FF, et al. The cochlear implant: historical aspects and future prospects. Anat Rec (Hoboken) 2012;295(11):1967–80.
4. Cochlear implants. 2017. Available at: https://www.nidcd.nih.gov/health/cochlear-implants. Accessed August 30, 2019.
5. Kalin R, Stanton MS. Current clinical issues for MRI scanning of pacemaker and defibrillator patients. Pacing Clin Electrophysiol 2005;28(4):326–8.
6. Heller JW, Brackmann DE, Tucci DL, et al. Evaluation of MRI compatibility of the modified nucleus multichannel auditory brainstem and cochlear implants. Am J Otol 1996;17(5):724–9.
7. Weber BP, Goldring JE, Santogrossi T, et al. Magnetic resonance imaging compatibility testing of the clarion 1.2 cochlear implant. Am J Otol 1998;19(5):584–90.

8. Teissl C, Kremser C, Hochmair ES, et al. Magnetic resonance imaging and cochlear implants: compatibility and safety aspects. J Magn Reson Imaging 1999;9(1):26–38.

9. Azadarmaki R, Tubbs R, Chen DA, et al. MRI information for commonly used otologic implants: review and update. Otolaryngol Head Neck Surg 2014;150(4): 512–9.

10. Pross SE, Ward BK, Sharon JD, et al. A prospective study of pain from magnetic resonance imaging with cochlear implant magnets in situ. Otol Neurotol 2018; 39(2):e80–6.

11. Crane BT, Gottschalk B, Kraut M, et al. Magnetic resonance imaging at 1.5 T after cochlear implantation. Otol Neurotol 2010;31(8):1215–20.

12. Walton J, Donnelly NP, Tam YC, et al. MRI without magnet removal in neurofibromatosis type 2 patients with cochlear and auditory brainstem implants. Otol Neurotol 2014;35(5):821–5.

13. Carlson ML, Neff BA, Link MJ, et al. Magnetic resonance imaging with cochlear implant magnet in place: safety and imaging quality. Otol Neurotol 2015;36(6): 965–71.

14. Kim BG, Kim JW, Park JJ, et al. Adverse events and discomfort during magnetic resonance imaging in cochlear implant recipients. JAMA Otolaryngol Head Neck Surg 2015;141(1):45–52.

15. Grupe G, Wagner J, Hofmann S, et al. Prevalence and complications of MRI scans of cochlear implant patients: English version. HNO 2017;65(Suppl 1): 35–40.

16. Takahashi D, Ogura A, Hayashi N, et al. The safety of MR conditional cochlear implant at 1.5 tesla magnetic resonance imaging system. Nihon Hoshasen Gijutsu Gakkai Zasshi 2016;72(8):674–80.

17. Todt I, Tittel A, Ernst A, et al. Pain free 3 T MRI scans in cochlear implantees. Otol Neurotol 2017;38(10):e401–4.

18. Todt I, Rademacher G, Mittmann P, et al. Postoperative imaging of the internal auditory canal: visualization of active auditory implants. HNO 2017;65(Suppl 2):81–6.

19. Sharon JD, Northcutt BG, Aygun N, et al. Magnetic resonance imaging at 1.5 tesla with a cochlear implant magnet in place: image quality and usability. Otol Neurotol 2016;37(9):1284–90.

20. Ralston A, Stevens G, Mahomudally E, et al. Cochlear implants: response to therapeutic irradiation. Int J Radiat Oncol Biol Phys 1999;44(1):227–31.

21. Klenzner T, Lutterbach J, Aschendorff A, et al. The effect of large single radiation doses on cochlear implant function: implications for radiosurgery. Eur Arch Otorhinolaryngol 2004;261(5):251–5.

22. Advanced Bionics L. INSTRUCTIONS FOR USE HiResolution™ bionic ear system. Manufacturer-provided instructions manual. Personal communication. June 25, 2018.

23. MED-EL. Medical procedures for MED-EL implant system. Available at: https://s3. medel.com/documents/AW/AW33289_30_Manual%20Medical%20Procedures% 20-%20EN%20English_web.pdf. Accessed July 8, 2019.

24. Manning C. Cochlear 2019. Manufacturer-provided information.

25. Maisel W, FDA. Programmable CSF shunts and magnetic field interference with implanted hearing devices - letter to health care providers 2019. Available at: https:// www.fda.gov/medical-devices/letters-health-care-providers/programmable-csf-shunts-and-magnetic-field-interference-implanted-hearing-devices-letter-health-care. Accessed July 16, 2019.

26. Wiet RM, El-Kashlan HK. Cochlear implantation in the presence of a programmable ventriculoperitoneal shunt. Otol Neurotol 2009;30(6):704–7.
27. An YH, Song SJ, Yoon SW, et al. Cochlear implantation for total deafness after ipsilateral ventriculoperitoneal shunt surgery: technical report. Acta Neurochir (Wien) 2011;153(12):247–83 [discussion: 2483].
28. Triglia JM, Beliaeff M, Faugere G. Cochlear implantation in a pacemaker patient. Laryngoscope 1996;106(9 Pt 1):1184–6.
29. Celenk F, Cevizci R, Altinyay S, et al. Cochlear implantation in extraordinary cases. Balkan Med J 2015;32(2):208–13.
30. St Martin MB, Hirsch BE. Cochlear implantation in a patient with bilateral deep brain stimulators. Laryngoscope 2007;117(1):183–5.
31. Shew M, Bertsch J, Camarata P, et al. Magnetic resonance imaging in a neurofibromatosis type 2 patient with a novel MRI-compatible auditory brainstem implant. J Neurol Surg Rep 2017;78(1):e12–4.
32. Certal VF, Zaghi S, Riaz M, et al. Hypoglossal nerve stimulation in the treatment of obstructive sleep apnea: a systematic review and meta-analysis. Laryngoscope 2015;125(5):1254–64.
33. Inspire Medical Systems I. MRI guidelines for inspire therapy. 2018. Available at: http://manuals.inspiresleep.com/wp-content/uploads/2018/05/200-261-101_EN_Rev-C_MRI-Guidelines_USA-only_eLABEL.pdf. Accessed August 30, 2019.
34. Vasconcellos AP, Huntley CT, Schell AE, et al. Dysfunctional hypoglossal nerve stimulator after electrical cardioversion: a case series. Laryngoscope 2019;129(8):1949–53.
35. Mingo K, Kominsky A. Electroconvulsive therapy for depression in a patient with an inspire hypoglossal nerve stimulator device for obstructive sleep apnea: a case report. Am J Otolaryngol 2018;39(4):462–3.
36. Patel SH, Halpern CH, Shepherd TM, et al. Electrical stimulation and monitoring devices of the CNS: an imaging review. J Neuroradiol 2017;44(3):175–84.
37. Thornton JS. Technical challenges and safety of magnetic resonance imaging with in situ neuromodulation from spine to brain. Eur J Paediatr Neurol 2017;21(1):232–41.
38. Rosch J, Hamer HM, Mennecke A, et al. 3T-MRI in patients with pharmacoresistant epilepsy and a vagus nerve stimulator: a pilot study. Epilepsy Res 2015;110:62–70.
39. Della Santina C. Vestibular implants 2019. Personal communication.
40. Holbrook EH, Puram SV, See RB, et al. Induction of smell through transethmoid electrical stimulation of the olfactory bulb. Int Forum Allergy Rhinol 2019;9(2):158–64.

Cranial Nerve Stimulation for Olfaction (Cranial Nerve 1)

Eric H. Holbrook, MD[a],*, Daniel H. Coelho, MD[b]

KEYWORDS

- Smell • Restoration • Implant • Electrode • Olfactory bulb

KEY POINTS

- Animal models support electrical stimulation of olfactory networks.
- Human electrical stimulation of the olfactory bulb stimulates smell.
- Olfactory electrical implants are feasible for restoring the sense of smell.

INTRODUCTION

Olfaction, or the sense of smell, plays a critical role in how people perceive and respond to their surroundings. Its role goes far beyond the enjoyment of odors or foods, because olfaction is important for the detection of potential dangers (eg, toxins, smoke, gas, spoiled food). Likewise, the sense of smell helps with social information, and is intimately associated with memory, cognition, and mood. Olfactory decline has been shown to portend neurologic disease and even preindicate death.[1] Many of the benefits that come with such an extraordinary sense are largely taken for granted until they are lost. As such, the loss of smell can have serious and long-lasting negative impacts on those who experience it. Therefore, any successful treatment would represent a much sought-after and long-overdue option for this challenging patient population. Although most treatments of sensorineural dysfunction have failed to effectively restore olfactory perception, recent promising advances in neurostimulation may represent a new era in the treatment of anosmia.

PATHOPHYSIOLOGY

Olfactory dysfunction can be characterized as either quantitative or qualitative. Quantitative dysfunction, by far the most common type of dysfunction, refers to the

Funding: D.H. Coelho's work on this article was partially funded through a grant from The MEDARVA Foundation, PT108029.
[a] Department of Otolaryngology Head & Neck Surgery, Massachusetts Eye & Ear, Harvard Medical School, 243 Charles Street, Boston, MA 02114, USA; [b] Department of Otolaryngology–Head & Neck Surgery, Virginia Commonwealth University School of Medicine, PO Box 980146, Richmond, VA 23298-0146, USA
* Corresponding author.
E-mail address: eric_holbrook@meei.harvard.edu

diminished or absent ability to detect odors and can range from normal (normosmic) to diminished (hyposmic) to absent (anosmic). Anosmia can also be specific to a particular class of odorants. Qualitative dysfunction (dysosmia) refers to altered perception of odorants, including parosmia and phantosmia. Parosmia is the distorted perception (usually unpleasant) in the presence of an odor source, whereas phantosmia refers to the persistent false perception of smell without an odor source, so it cannot be masked by other odorants.

Like hearing loss, olfactory dysfunction can also be described as either congenital or acquired. Almost all cases are acquired, because the incidence of congenital anosmia is estimated to range from 1 in 5000 to 1 in 10,000.[2] Also like hearing loss, olfactory pathophysiology can be thought of as conductive (peripheral) or sensorineural (central). Conductive loss comes from any process that mechanically blocks the flow of odorant delivery to the olfactory receptors within the olfactory cleft nasal mucosa. These processes include obstructive nasal diseases such as chronic rhinosinusitis, nasal polyposis, septal deviations, allergic rhinitis, and nasal masses. These conditions are generally amenable to medical or surgical treatment, and with restoration of airflow and odorant delivery comes improved olfaction. Sensorineural smell loss occurs within the neural substrate of the olfactory pathway, thereby impairing or completely blocking the transmission of signal to the brain. The site of injury can be anywhere from the olfactory receptor nerves to the olfactory cortex. The most common causes of such loss are postinfectious (viral), posttraumatic, postsurgical, toxic, age related, neurodegenerative (ie, Parkinson, Alzheimer), and idiopathic.

EPIDEMIOLOGY

Determining the exact number of people who have olfactory disorders has proved difficult. Self-reported prevalence ranges from approximately 1.4% to 15.3%.[3] Although similar to the range of prevalence of 2.7% to 24.5% that has been reported in several objective, population-based studies, self-reporting generally underestimates olfactory impairment.[3] For anosmia, or the complete loss of smell, far fewer data are available. In their study of 1387 Swedish volunteers, Nordin and colleagues[4] report a 5.8% prevalence of anosmia. In their study of nearly 10,000 people in Catalonia, Spain, Mullol and colleagues[5] found only a 0.3% prevalence of anosmia. However, they based their findings on the subjective, unconfirmed ability to detect odorants microencapsulated in a daily newspaper.[5] Recent nationally representative data reveal that anosmia afflicts 3.2% of US adults who are aged more than 40 years (3.4 million people) and this number increases with age (14%–22% of those aged 60 years and older).[6–8] With consideration given to the difficulty in providing an exact number of people afflicted with anosmia, a recent consensus reviewing current literature estimates a prevalence of approximately 5% of the general population[9]

Most of the epidemiologic data on anosmia come from the head injury literature.[10] The first reports appear in the late 1800s, when the cases of anosmia are mostly attributed to falls from horses or blows to the head.[11] The earliest estimates of anosmia following head injury suggested an incidence of 4% to 7%, although these reports varied widely in severity of injury as well as the methods used to assess the dysfunction.[12,13] In their 1991 review, Costanzo and Zasler[14] reported anosmia in 25% to 30% of patients with severe head injury, 15% to 19% of those with moderate head injury, and 0% to 16% of those with mild injuries. Other, but not all, subsequent studies have reported similar correlations between severity of injury and degree of olfactory dysfunction.[15–18]

The prevalence of phantosmia (the persistent false perception of smell that cannot be masked by other odorants) is estimated between 0.8% and 2.1%.[19] Parosmia (the distorted perception, unusually unpleasant, in the presence of an odor source) is found in approximately 4% of patients with abnormal olfaction.[4] These distortions of smell severely magnify the detriment in quality of life already experienced by those with smell loss.[20] For an excellent review of the epidemiology of olfactory disorders, readers are referred to Yang and Pinto.[3]

QUALITY OF LIFE IN ANOSMIA

Loss of smell, despite its innocuous presentation, can have devastating long-term effects, long after the initial insults have resolved or stabilized. In disability calculation, The American Medical Association impairment ratings suggest a "5% impairment of a whole person" for those with bilateral anosmia (unilateral loss has no associated impairment).[21] However, this does not necessarily correlate to the degree of the patients' subjective impairment, which can be debilitating, particularly in patients whose vocations depend greatly on their ability to smell; for example, chefs, chemists, plumbers, firefighters, florists, cosmeticians. Anosmia is negatively correlated with successful vocational reintegration, although this may also be caused by associated neurocognitive dysfunction.

There are many other adverse effects of smell loss that affect activities of daily living (ADLs), quality of life, safety, appetite, nutrition, hygiene, homemaking, childcare, and hobbies. In their 2001 retrospective study of 420 patients (345 of whom complained of substantial impairment of ADLs), Miwa and colleagues[22] characterized the most commonly cited activities impaired by olfactory dysfunction. The 2 most common adverse effects (spoiled food, gas detection) involve personal safety and must be discussed with patients. Dating of perishable food items, and proper installation and maintenance of smoke and gas detectors in the home, are strongly advised. Santos and colleagues[23] reported at least 1 hazardous event in 45.2% of patients with anosmia, 34.1% with severe hyposmia, 32.8% with moderate hyposmia, and 24.2% with mild hyposmia. However, the authors found that 19.0% of patients with normal olfactory testing had at least 1 hazardous event. Risk of hazardous events seems to be statistically higher in women, patients more than 65 years of age, and African Americans.[24]

Patients must also be counseled on cooking and nutrition, because olfactory dysfunction greatly impairs the appreciation and tolerance of food, even leading to food aversion in some cases of parosmia. Some patients seek to compensate for loss of flavor perception by adding salty, sweet, crunchy, or spicy food to their diets, which stimulates intact trigeminal or chorda tympani pathways. However, some of these supplements may themselves have negative effects on nutrition and health.[25,26] Beyond the risks to health, patients with diminished smell may have problems with personal hygiene, child care, and pet care. Patients should be made aware of this potential, and schedules should be firmly established.

People with intact olfaction seldom carefully consider the impact of not being able to enjoy the flavor of a favorite meal, the smell of morning coffee, or the scents of a child or partner. However, for those afflicted with loss of smell, quality of life is greatly impaired. Numerous studies have shown strong relationships between olfactory disturbances and clinical depression.[27] In Miwa and colleagues'[22] study, 50% of all patients with impaired olfaction reported being either very or somewhat satisfied with life, with 45% reporting being either very or somewhat dissatisfied with life.[22] Because the sense of smell is intimately associated with mood, cognition, and memory, deterioration in these domains is frequently seen in patients with anosmia. However, any successful intervention to address anosmia has a significant positive influence on these same domains.

CURRENT STATE OF MANAGEMENT

With consideration of the prevalence of olfactory dysfunction, the substantial impact on quality of life, and low likelihood of spontaneous recovery, it is discouraging that few effective treatments exist for this patient population. Patients with inflammatory causes of smell loss are the exception. In these cases, treatment of the underlying disease process typically provides substantial improvement through the use of corticosteroids in systemic and topical forms, frequently with the addition of surgery to aid in the ventilation of the paranasal sinuses and removal of obstructing polyps. However, inflammatory causes of smell loss are only a fraction of all causes. In conditions such as upper respiratory infections, head trauma, and aging, treatments are few and have minimal effect. With regard to the use of systemic and topical medications, various studies have reported on the use of corticosteroids, phosphodiesterase inhibitors, intranasal calcium buffers, and other medications; however, insufficient evidence exists relating to the efficacy of these treatments for use in noninflammatory olfactory disorders.[9]

Unlike the pharmaceuticals mentioned earlier with limited evidence showing reproducible benefits in treating noninflammatory smell loss, the practice of olfactory training has been shown to provide benefits in multiple studies. Hummel and colleagues[28] first reported the benefits of smelling the odors of rose, eucalyptus, lemon, and clove twice daily for 3 months in patients with multiple causes of olfactory loss. Subsequent studies have shown greater improvements with stronger odors and longer duration of treatment.[29] However, despite the repeated evidence for improvement, this training technique has limitations and a treatment providing wholesale reversal of olfactory loss continues to be elusive.

Although current available treatments are lacking, recent research efforts to address neuronal injury to the olfactory nerves have shown some promise. In a mouse model, Kobayashi and Costanzo[30] showed that treatment with steroids improves recovery outcome following olfactory nerve injury. In addition, blockage of specific pathways mediating the inflammatory response could also provide a new strategy for the treatment of posttraumatic olfactory dysfunction. Interleukin-6 reduces astrocyte and macrophage levels in the areas of olfactory injury and contributes to improved olfactory nerve regeneration and recovery.[31] Other approaches to repair and restoration of olfactory function involve the grafting or transplant of olfactory epithelial tissue to sites of injury. Chen and colleagues[32] transplanted olfactory progenitor cells into the olfactory epithelium of mice after chemical injury and showed that the progenitor cells gave rise to globose basal cells, neurons, and sustentacular cells. Isolating and growing olfactory basal stem cells in culture provides a model for understanding the regulation of neuronal regeneration.[33–35] Recently, the ability to isolate and expand the horizontal basal cells obtained from human olfactory epithelium and push them toward neuronal differentiation has been reported, setting the stage for potential stem cell therapies.[36]

Despite scientific advances in understanding the mechanisms involved in regeneration of olfactory neurons and the pathophysiology of smell loss, therapeutic breakthroughs in olfactory disorders are lagging. However, patients with anosmia should not lose hope. Recent developments in neurostimulation have shown great promise.

STIMULATION OF CRANIAL NERVE 1

As with all aspects of olfaction, clinical research and treatment lag behind those of many other cranial nerve deficits (eg, hearing loss, vision). However, recent discoveries in olfactory physiology have improved the understanding of smell, and likewise have paved the way for some potentially novel therapeutic options. Such advances are based largely on improved understanding of olfactory functional architecture, providing the groundwork for electrical stimulation to restore the sense of smell.

The sense of smell begins with the presentation of odors to the olfactory epithelium within the nasal cavity. Here odorants bind to receptors on olfactory sensory neurons (OSNs), resulting in transduction into electrical signals. Each of the 15 million OSNs in the mouse expresses only 1 type of odorant receptor gene.[37–39] Axons of OSNs that share the same odorant receptor-type project through the cribriform plate, enter into the olfactory bulb, and converge on a few localized glomeruli.[40–42] It is among these glomeruli and olfactory bulb mitral cells that the spatial patterns of neural activity encode odor identity and intensity and constitute the basis of an odor map[43–45] (**Fig. 1**). This organizational map seems to be preserved with projections to higher centers. Early electrophysiology experiments showed spatial unit responses in the thalamus of rabbits and lateral habenular nucleus in rats after electrical stimulation of the olfactory bulb.[46,47] Further studies with neuronal tracers have shown topographic projections from different regions of the olfactory bulb to specific areas of the anterior

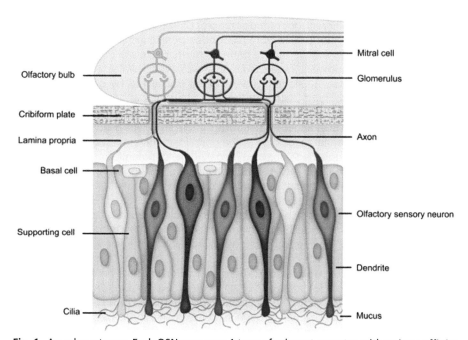

Fig. 1. An odorant map. Each OSN expresses 1 type of odorant receptor with unique affinity for various odorant chemicals. Within the olfactory epithelium, OSNs with like receptors are dispersed among other OSNs but their axons converge as they transverse the cribriform plate and make terminal synapses within glomeruli of the olfactory bulb. Each glomerulus contains the axon terminals from OSNs expressing the same odorant receptor; with exposure to an odor, a defined set of OSNs are activated that in turn activate a subset of glomeruli within the olfactory bulb. (*From* C. Trimmer, J.D. Mainland. The Olfactory System. Conn's Translational Neuroscience 2017; 363–377; with permission.)

olfactory nucleus.[48] These specific projections to the anterior olfactory nucleus seem to be functionally relevant based on cFos activity in response to odor presentation and electrical stimulation of the olfactory bulb.[49]

The spatial organization within special sensory pathways is not unique to olfaction. Within otolaryngology, the tonotopic organization of the cochlea is perhaps the most well known and has been capitalized on with substantial success in the case of cochlear implants for the treatment of sensorineural hearing loss. By stimulating different areas of the cochlea with varying currents and with different time intervals and patterns, cochlear implants have been able to restore near-normal sound perception in deaf patients. Likewise, by using the same principles of highly focused patterns of electrical stimulation to the olfactory bulb, unique smell perceptions theoretically could be achieved.

When OSNs and their nerve fibers are damaged and normal neural impulses cannot be transmitted to the olfactory bulb, direct electrical stimulation of the olfactory bulb can be used to generate patterns of neural activity. These patterns of activity in the bulb, similar to normal olfactory processing, could theoretically lead to the perception of smell (providing that the cause of anosmia did not disrupt olfactory bulb anatomy or physiology). This possibility was shown by Coelho and Costanzo,[50] who used both odors and electrical stimulation of the olfactory bulb in rats to show the spatial mapping of neural responses in the olfactory bulb. They analyzed multiunit responses to odor stimulation and evoked potential responses to localized electrical stimulation measured in different regions of the olfactory bulb, showing different spatial patterns of neural activity for different odors (odor maps). Direct stimulation of the olfactory bulb with electrical current pulses from electrodes positioned at different locations was also effective in generating spatial patterns of neural activity. Subsequent work in an animal model of anosmia (transected OSNs) was effective in generating localized field potential responses.[51] Olfactory nerves were transected by passing a Teflon blade between the cribriform plate and the ventral surface of the bulb. A cochlear implant electrode array was used to stimulate 6 different positions along the ventral surface of the olfactory bulb and a 16-electrode paddle array was used to record localized negative field potential responses at the dorsal surface of the bulb (**Fig. 2**). The investigators reliably obtained localized negative field potentials using biphasic, 500-μA, 200-microsecond pulses. A shift in stimulating position by 1 mm resulted in a significant change in the dorsal field potential, suggesting direct stimulation of the deafferented olfactory bulb is effective in generating localized field potential responses. In support of electrical stimulation generating true olfactory perception, Mouly and colleagues[52] trained rats using a water-deprivation model and showed the ability of the rats to distinguish electrical stimulation of the mitral cell layer even when electrodes were spatially separated by as little as 250 μm. These findings support the potential use of direct electrical stimulation for the treatment of anosmia in humans.

Electrical stimulation of human olfaction has been attempted in the past. Electrically reproducing a perception of smell through stimulating electrodes placed in the nasal cavity on the olfactory epithelium has not been reliable. Ishimaru and colleagues[53] were able to record evoked potentials from the ipsilateral frontal region during olfactory epithelium stimulation and Weiss and colleagues[54] noted activity in the piriform cortex based on functional MRI findings. Although patients did not report a sensation of smell, these studies suggest a progression of the electrical stimulus delivered at the olfactory epithelium to more central regions. In 1 study, 3 subjects with electric stimulation of the olfactory mucosa reported a sensation of smell; however, all 3 had a history of seizures with olfactory auras. In the same study, 2 subjects with epilepsy but

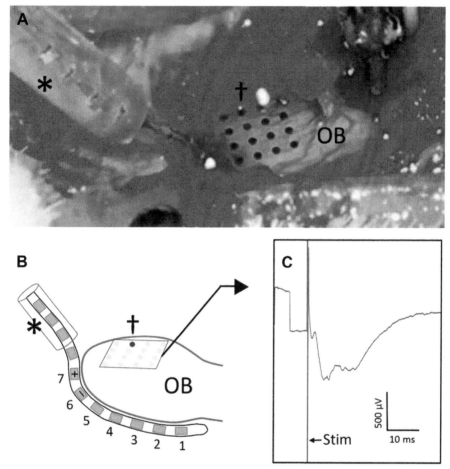

Fig. 2. (*A*) Cochlear implant–stimulating electrodes (*asterisk*) inserted under the rat olfactory bulb (OB) and a 4 × 4 array of surface recoding electrodes (*dagger*). (*B*) Location of the bipolar stimulus at electrodes 7 (+) and 6 (−) and surface recording electrode (*red dot*). (*C*) Negative evoked potential response. Calibration pulse appears before the stimulus artifact (Stim). (*Adapted from* Coelho DH, Socolovsky LD, Costanzo RM. Activation of the rat olfactory bulb by direct ventral stimulation after nerve transection. Int Forum Allergy Rhinol. May 2018. https://doi.org/10.1002/alr.22133; with permission.)

without olfactory auras did not perceive a smell with epithelial electrical stimulation.[55] It was concluded that the electrical stimulation was only triggering the epileptic auras. Although electrical stimulation of the epithelium has not shown convincing generation of a sensation of smell, electric stimulation of the olfactory bulb or surrounding brain structures has successfully produced an olfactory sensory perception. Penfield and Jasper[56] reported the regular ability to induce a smell during intraoperative electrode stimulation of the olfactory bulb in awake patients with epilepsy undergoing mapping for seizure control. They reported 1 patient who identified the smell as similar to "the manure pile over in the back lot near the short-cut."[56] More recently, olfactory hallucinations were stimulated in multiple children with epilepsy undergoing subdural electrode stimulation of ventral frontal lobe, which is in proximity to the olfactory bulb. The investigators suggested that the stimulation was likely spreading to the olfactory bulb, resulting in the subjective smell perception.[57] Similarly, a recent study also reported sensation of smell initiated by 6 of 651 electrical stimulations of the central sulcus of the insula when delivered to 221 patients with implanted electrodes for drug-refractory seizures.[58]

With these prior results in mind, Holbrook and colleagues[59] investigated the ability to induce a subjective perception of smell with transnasal electrical stimulation of the olfactory bulb through the thin bone of the cribriform plate. Five subjects with a history of prior sinus surgery, including total ethmoidectomy, with intact ability to smell were enrolled. Awake subjects underwent nasal endoscopy and stimulating electrodes were positioned at 3 areas along the lateral lamella of the cribriform plate within the ethmoid sinus cavity. Graded stimulation currents from 1 to 20 mA at 3.17 Hz were administered while cortical evoked potential (CEP) recordings were collected. Although CEP recordings correlating with olfaction were not reliably detected, 3 subjects reported a perception of a smell with electrical stimulation. In addition, the electrical induction of a smell was reproducible even after applying lidocaine to the olfactory epithelium in order to produce a temporary anosmia. This finding added further evidence that the electrical stimulation in this paradigm was bypassing the olfactory epithelium and activating neurons within the olfactory bulb.

FUTURE DIRECTIONS

Although electrostimulation of the human olfactory system is in its infancy (compared with cochlear implantation), the development of one such olfactory implant system (OIS) is already underway. First described by Coelho and Costanzo[50] at Virginia Commonwealth University School of Medicine (US Patent 9517342B2), the OIS is composed of 4 main components: a sensor array, a microprocessor, a transmitter/receiver, and an electrode array (**Fig. 3**). The sensor array is similar to those commonly used in so-called electronic noses. Electronic noses have traditionally been used in the industrial and manufacturing sectors, but are now seen more commonly in the

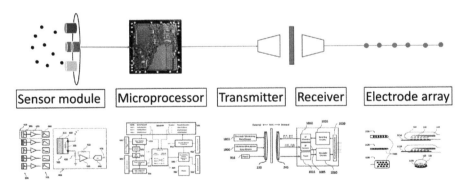

Fig. 3. Components of the OIS (US patent 9,517,342).[2] The OIS is composed of 4 main components: a sensor array module, a microprocessor, a transmitter/receiver, and an electrode array. The sensor array is similar to those used in electronic noses. The sensor array is used to generate unique digital fingerprints (odor fingerprint) for a given smell. The microprocessor matches odor fingerprints with programmed electrode stimulation patterns known to elicit specific odor perceptions. The stimulation patterns are transmitted to a receiver that provides current pulses to the electrode array for direct stimulation of the olfactory bulb.

biomedical and health care fields. A variety of sensor technologies are currently available, including metal-oxide semiconductors, polymer conductors, polymer composites, quartz crystal microbalancers, surface acoustic waves, ultrafast mass gas chromatography, and mass spectrometry. Combinations of these have allowed even more fine discrimination of odors. More recently, bioelectronic noses have been developed by coating human olfactory receptors on field effect transistor devices that theoretically more closely mimic the sense of smell.[60–62] Irrespective of the individual technology used or whether single or multiple sensors are used, sensors can be used to generate unique digital fingerprints (odor fingerprint) for a given smell.

In the OIS, the odor fingerprint is then transmitted to a microprocessor where it is matched with the appropriate stimulating pattern. Like a cochlear implant, the processor then sends the stimulating pattern to the transmitter, which in turns sends the signal transcutaneously to the implanted receiver/stimulator. From there the electrode array at the olfactory bulb is stimulated according the appropriate pattern. The electrode array is shaped to conform to the ventral surface of the olfactory bulb. Efforts to determine the ideal method of surgical implantation and transcutaneous signal transfer are ongoing.

Optimizing the appropriate stimulating pattern for a given odor fingerprint will require mapping sessions. During these sessions, the implanted array is stimulated in a variety of different ways (eg, number and location of electrodes stimulated, current, pulse width, phase). Experience in cochlear implantation and the ability to exquisitely tune external auditory signals into nuanced electrical stimulation will certainly be a rich source of prior experience that could be applied to olfaction. The patients will then be asked to report which smell is most closely approximated by that stimulating pattern. The response is then linked to the odor fingerprint for that smell. That link is saved within the memory of the microprocessor, so that on subsequent exposure to that smell the same stimulating pattern will be used, resulting in a perception of smell that is unique and repeatable.

This system has limitations. Despite major advances in the abilities of odor sensor technology, sensors currently cannot identify each of the estimated 1 trillion unique smells discernible by the human olfactory system.[63] However, that estimate is based on combinations of multiple unique odorants per smell and the quantification of every odorant may not be necessary to properly identify the smell. For example, the scent of a rose is composed of a mixture of 275 unique odorants, although only a very small percentage of those odorants are necessary for its identification.[64] The OI system processor would therefore need to store hundreds, and not trillions, of odor fingerprint profiles in its memory. In contrast, the number of electrodes and variable modes of their stimulation could conceivably create novel perceptions of smell even in the absence of odorant input.

Current limitations in electrode array design, size, and layout may not allow the resolution necessary for fine discriminations of smell. However, as has been learned from cochlear implantation, the pattern of electrode stimulation may play a much more important role than the number or configuration of electrodes. In addition, it is unlikely that the mitral/glomerular organization of smell is fixed from person to person. Even if it was, the size of the olfactory bulb differs from person to person, and the ability to consistently and precisely place an electrode array would pose a significant technical challenge. As a result, this system relies on subjective association and recall postimplantation and may not be appropriate for adults with congenital anosmia. Preclinical safety testing is expected to begin in 2020.

Even in the early stages, the OIS has already garnered significant interest across the clinical, scientific, business, and lay populations. In their 2018 article, Besser and colleagues[65] suggested that, among patients with olfactory dysfunction, olfactory implants would be of great interest, with more than 34% of patients indicating an openness to trying such technology, even when they are aware that such a procedure may involve head surgery using a neurosurgical approach. First-in-human trials are still years away, but all indications point to a device that could become the first viable treatment of patients with anosmia. Over time, other nonolfactory benefits to cognition, mood, and memory may prove to be the major applications of this technology. Fortunately, the substantial knowledge gained in the development of nonolfactory cranial nerve stimulation (particular cochlear implantation) provides a deep well of technical knowledge from which to draw.

SUMMARY

There is a clear unmet need for a treatment directed toward the millions of patients with loss of smell. As with other sensory systems, a concerted effort along parallel pathways directed toward development of therapies to restore smell should be supported. In addition to trials using existing medications, the development of new pharmacologic agents, as well as manipulation of olfactory epithelium stem cells; artificial stimulation of the olfactory system deserves equal attention. Olfactory researchers should take note of this similar approach adopted by investigators in other sensory systems. Prior studies and recent advances in technology support the rationale for efforts directed toward artificial stimulation. The high prevalence of afflicted patients without smell and the documented negative effect on quality of life underscore the need for continued development of such novel therapeutics.

DISCLOSURE

D.H. Coelho has equity in Lawnboy Ventures, LLC. E.H. Holbrook has nothing to disclose.

REFERENCES

1. Shepherd GM. The human sense of smell: are we better than we think? PLoS Biol 2004;2(5):E146.
2. Croy I, Negoias S, Novakova L, et al. Learning about the functions of the olfactory system from people without a sense of smell. PLoS One 2012;7(3):e33365.
3. Yang J, Pinto JM. The epidemiology of olfactory disorders. Curr Otorhinolaryngol Rep 2016;4(2):130–41.
4. Nordin S, Brämerson A, Millqvist E, et al. Prevalence of parosmia: the Skövde population-based studies. Rhinology 2007;45(1):50–3.
5. Mullol J, Alobid I, Mariño-Sánchez F, et al. Furthering the understanding of olfaction, prevalence of loss of smell and risk factors: a population-based survey (OLFACAT study). BMJ Open 2012;2(6). https://doi.org/10.1136/bmjopen-2012-001256.
6. Kern DW, Wroblewski KE, Schumm LP, et al. Olfactory function in wave 2 of the National Social Life, Health, and Aging Project. J Gerontol B Psychol Sci Soc Sci 2014;69(Suppl 2):S134–43.
7. Pinto JM, Wroblewski KE, Kern DW, et al. Olfactory dysfunction predicts 5-year mortality in older adults. PLoS One 2014;9(10):e107541.
8. Hoffman HJ, Ishii EK, MacTurk RH. Age-related changes in the prevalence of smell/taste problems among the United States adult population. Results of the

1994 disability supplement to the National Health Interview Survey (NHIS). Ann N Y Acad Sci 1998;855:716–22.

9. Hummel T, Whitcroft KL, Andrews P, et al. Position paper on olfactory dysfunction. Rhinol Suppl 2017;54(26):1–30.

10. Coelho DH, Costanzo RM. Posttraumatic olfactory dysfunction. Auris Nasus Larynx 2016;43(2):137–43.

11. Legg JW. A case of anosmia following a blow. Lancet 1873;102(2619):659–60.

12. Leigh AD. Defects of smell after head injury. Lancet 1943;241(6228):38–40.

13. Kraus JF, Fife D, Ramstein K, et al. The relationship of family income to the incidence, external causes, and outcomes of serious brain injury, San Diego County, California. Am J Public Health 1986;76(11):1345–7.

14. Costanzo RM, Zasler N. Head trauma. In: Getchell TV, editor. Smell and taste in health and disease. New York: Raven Press; 1991. p. 711–30.

15. Cain WS. Testing olfaction in a clinical setting. Ear Nose Throat J 1989;68(4):316, 322–328.

16. Ikeda K, Tabata K, Oshima T, et al. Unilateral examination of olfactory threshold using the Jet Stream Olfactometer. Auris Nasus Larynx 1999;26(4):435–9.

17. Kondo H, Matsuda T, Hashiba M, et al. A study of the relationship between the T&T olfactometer and the University of Pennsylvania Smell Identification Test in a Japanese population. Am J Rhinol 1998;12(5):353–8.

18. Fortin A, Lefebvre MB, Ptito M. Traumatic brain injury and olfactory deficits: the tale of two smell tests! Brain Inj 2010;24(1):27–33.

19. Landis BN, Konnerth CG, Hummel T. A study on the frequency of olfactory dysfunction. Laryngoscope 2004;114(10):1764–9.

20. Bonfils P, Avan P, Faulcon P, et al. Distorted odorant perception: analysis of a series of 56 patients with parosmia. Arch Otolaryngol Head Neck Surg 2005;131(2): 107–12.

21. Rondinelli RD. Changes for the new AMA Guides to impairment ratings, 6th edition: implications and applications for physician disability evaluations. PM R 2009;1(7):643–56. Available at: https://www.ncbi.nlm.nih.gov/pubmed/ 19627958. Accessed May 7, 2019.

22. Miwa T, Furukawa M, Tsukatani T, et al. Impact of olfactory impairment on quality of life and disability. Arch Otolaryngol Head Neck Surg 2001;127(5):497–503.

23. Santos DV, Reiter ER, DiNardo LJ, et al. Hazardous events associated with impaired olfactory function. Arch Otolaryngol Head Neck Surg 2004;130(3): 317–9.

24. Pence TS, Reiter ER, DiNardo LJ, et al. Risk factors for hazardous events in olfactory-impaired patients. JAMA Otolaryngol Head Neck Surg 2014;140(10): 951–5.

25. Mattes RD, Cowart BJ. Dietary assessment of patients with chemosensory disorders. J Am Diet Assoc 1994;94(1):50–6.

26. Ferris AM, Duffy VB. Effect of olfactory deficits on nutritional status. Does age predict persons at risk? Ann N Y Acad Sci 1989;561:113–23.

27. Temmel AFP, Quint C, Schickinger-Fischer B, et al. Characteristics of olfactory disorders in relation to major causes of olfactory loss. Arch Otolaryngol Head Neck Surg 2002;128(6):635–41.

28. Hummel T, Rissom K, Reden J, et al. Effects of olfactory training in patients with olfactory loss. Laryngoscope 2009;119(3):496–9.

29. Damm M, Pikart LK, Reimann H, et al. Olfactory training is helpful in postinfectious olfactory loss: a randomized, controlled, multicenter study. Laryngoscope 2014;124(4):826–31.

30. Kobayashi M, Costanzo RM. Olfactory nerve recovery following mild and severe injury and the efficacy of dexamethasone treatment. Chem Senses 2009;34(7): 573–80.

31. Kobayashi M, Tamari K, Miyamura T, et al. Blockade of interleukin-6 receptor suppresses inflammatory reaction and facilitates functional recovery following olfactory system injury. Neurosci Res 2013;76(3):125–32.

32. Chen X, Fang H, Schwob JE. Multipotency of purified, transplanted globose basal cells in olfactory epithelium. J Comp Neurol 2004;469(4):457–74.

33. Jang W, Lambropoulos J, Woo JK, et al. Maintaining epitheliopoietic potency when culturing olfactory progenitors. Exp Neurol 2008;214(1):25–36.

34. Goldstein BJ, Goss GM, Choi R, et al. Contribution of Polycomb group proteins to olfactory basal stem cell self-renewal in a novel c-KIT+ culture model and in vivo. Development 2016;143(23):4394–404.

35. Schwob JE, Jang W, Holbrook EH, et al. Stem and progenitor cells of the mammalian olfactory epithelium: taking poietic license. J Comp Neurol 2017;525(4): 1034–54.

36. Peterson J, Lin B, Barrios-Camacho CM, et al. Activating a reserve neural stem cell population in vitro enables engraftment and multipotency after transplantation. Stem Cell Rep 2019;12(4):680–95.

37. Duchamp-Viret P, Duchamp A, Chaput MA. Peripheral odor coding in the rat and frog: quality and intensity specification. J Neurosci 2000;20(6):2383–90.

38. Malnic B, Hirono J, Sato T, et al. Combinatorial receptor codes for odors. Cell 1999;96(5):713–23.

39. Buck L, Axel R. A novel multigene family may encode odorant receptors: a molecular basis for odor recognition. Cell 1991;65(1):175–87.

40. Mombaerts P. Targeting olfaction. Curr Opin Neurobiol 1996;6(4):481–6.

41. Mombaerts P, Wang F, Dulac C, et al. Visualizing an olfactory sensory map. Cell 1996;87(4):675–86.

42. Serizawa S, Ishii T, Nakatani H, et al. Mutually exclusive expression of odorant receptor transgenes. Nat Neurosci 2000;3(7):687–93.

43. Rubin BD, Katz LC. Optical imaging of odorant representations in the mammalian olfactory bulb. Neuron 1999;23(3):499–511.

44. Uchida N, Takahashi YK, Tanifuji M, et al. Odor maps in the mammalian olfactory bulb: domain organization and odorant structural features. Nat Neurosci 2000; 3(10):1035–43.

45. Belluscio L, Katz LC. Symmetry, stereotypy, and topography of odorant representations in mouse olfactory bulbs. J Neurosci 2001;21(6):2113–22.

46. Jackson JC, Benjamin RM. Unit discharges in the mediodorsal nucleus of the rabbit evoked by electrical stimulation of the olfactory bulb. Brain Res 1974; 75(2):193–201.

47. Mok AC, Mogenson GJ. Effects of electrical stimulation of the lateral hypothalamus, hippocampus, amygdala and olfactory bulb on unit activity of the lateral habenular nucleus in the rat. Brain Res 1974;77(3):417–29.

48. Yan Z, Tan J, Qin C, et al. Precise circuitry links bilaterally symmetric olfactory maps. Neuron 2008;58(4):613–24.

49. Kay RB, Meyer EA, Illig KR, et al. Spatial distribution of neural activity in the anterior olfactory nucleus evoked by odor and electrical stimulation. J Comp Neurol 2011;519(2):277–89.

50. Coelho DH, Costanzo RM. Spatial mapping in the rat olfactory bulb by odor and direct electrical stimulation. Otolaryngol Head Neck Surg 2016;155(3):526–32.

51. Coelho DH, Socolovsky LD, Costanzo RM. Activation of the rat olfactory bulb by direct ventral stimulation after nerve transection. Int Forum Allergy Rhinol 2018. https://doi.org/10.1002/alr.22133.
52. Mouly AM, Vigouroux M, Holley A. On the ability of rats to discriminate between microstimulations of the olfactory bulb in different locations. Behav Brain Res 1985;17(1):45–58.
53. Ishimaru T, Shimada T, Sakumoto M, et al. Olfactory evoked potential produced by electrical stimulation of the human olfactory mucosa. Chem Senses 1997; 22(1):77–81.
54. Weiss T, Shushan S, Ravia A, et al. From nose to brain: un-sensed electrical currents applied in the nose alter activity in deep brain structures. Cereb Cortex 2016. https://doi.org/10.1093/cercor/bhw222.
55. Straschill M, Stahl H, Gorkisch K. Effects of electrical stimulation of the human olfactory mucosa. Appl Neurophysiol 1983;46(5–6):286–9.
56. Penfield W, Jasper H. Epilepsy and the functional anatomy of the human brain. Boston: Little, Brown and Co.; 1954.
57. Kumar G, Juhász C, Sood S, et al. Olfactory hallucinations elicited by electrical stimulation via subdural electrodes: effects of direct stimulation of olfactory bulb and tract. Epilepsy Behav 2012;24(2):264–8.
58. Mazzola L, Royet J-P, Catenoix H, et al. Gustatory and olfactory responses to stimulation of the human insula. Ann Neurol 2017;82(3):360–70.
59. Holbrook EH, Puram SV, See RB, et al. Induction of smell through transethmoid electrical stimulation of the olfactory bulb. Int Forum Allergy Rhinol 2019;9(2): 158–64.
60. Goldsmith BR, Mitala JJ, Josue J, et al. Biomimetic chemical sensors using nanoelectronic readout of olfactory receptor proteins. ACS Nano 2011;5(7):5408–16.
61. Ko HJ, Lee SH, Oh EH, et al. Specificity of odorant-binding proteins: a factor influencing the sensitivity of olfactory receptor-based biosensors. Bioproc Biosyst Eng 2010;33(1):55–62.
62. Yoon H, Lee SH, Kwon OS, et al. Polypyrrole nanotubes conjugated with human olfactory receptors: high-performance transducers for FET-type bioelectronic noses. Angew Chem Int Ed Engl 2009;48(15):2755–8.
63. Bushdid C, Magnasco MO, Vosshall LB, et al. Humans can discriminate more than 1 trillion olfactory stimuli. Science 2014;343(6177):1370–2.
64. Ohloff G. The fascination of odors and their chemical perspectives. Berlin: Springer-Verlag; 1994.
65. Besser G, Liu DT, Renner B, et al. Olfactory implant: demand for a future treatment option in patients with olfactory dysfunction. Laryngoscope 2019;129(2): 312–6.

Cochlear Implant

James G. Naples, MD[a],*, Michael J. Ruckenstein, MD[b]

KEYWORDS

- Cochlear implantation • Hearing loss • Implantable hearing device
- Neural stimulation

KEY POINTS

- Cochlear implant is the first effective cranial nerve stimulator. It revolutionized management of permanent sensorineural hearing loss in adults and children.
- Indications for cochlear implant depend on detailed audiologic assessment and are evolving to offer implantation for patients with residual low frequency hearing.
- Outcomes for adult and pediatric cochlear implant patients are favorable and depend on various patient and procedural factors.
- Future advances in cochlear implant will be aimed at optimizing the interaction between the electrical stimuli and the cochlear nerve.

INTRODUCTION
Impact of Cochlear Implant

It is impossible to overstate the medical and societal impact of cochlear implant (CI). The introduction of this device allowed otolaryngologists to restore auditory input in deafened adult and pediatric patients. From a societal perspective, it offers prelingually deafened children and postlingually deafened adults the opportunity to reenter the hearing, social world. Similarly, it opens the door for children to integrate into the mainstream education system. Medically, it has changed the conversation for otolaryngologists on deafness, and introduced options for sensorineural hearing loss (SNHL) beyond amplification. In addition, the CI was the first successful implantable cranial nerve stimulator. There was significant risk in production of the CI, and skepticism was a theme in its early years. Fortunately, pioneers from the fields of otolaryngology, audiology, and engineering persevered and continued to push the limits of what was possible. As experience with this device grows, it has served as a prototype for newer cranial nerve implants by demonstrating that restoration of function is

Disclosure Statement: The authors have nothing to disclose.
[a] Division of Otolaryngology, Beth Israel Deaconess Medical Center, Harvard Medical School, 110 Francis St, Suite 6E, Boston, MA 02215; [b] Department of Otorhinolaryngology—Head and Neck Surgery, University of Pennsylvania Health System, 3400 Spruce Street, 5 Silverstein Philadelphia, PA 19104, USA
* Corresponding author.
E-mail address: Jnaples513@gmail.com

possible. It is extraordinary to understand how the early CI has evolved to its current state, and the evolution of this device has pushed the otolaryngology community to expect better outcomes for patients. We anticipate that the future concepts of stimulation of the cochlear nerve will continue to evolve and serve as a prototype for other implantable cranial nerve stimulators that have potential to restore essential functions for patients and have a positive social impact.

The Cochlear Implant Device

There are a variety of commercially available CI devices; however, the concept behind the hardware components of CI are similar among the various devices. In general, the hardware consists of (1) an external device that receives and processes the sounds and (2) and internal device that transduces the received signal and directly stimulates the cochlear nerve (**Fig. 1**). Although the concept behind the implant is simple, the production and execution of a prosthesis that restores sound input is exceedingly complex. As history has demonstrated, early attempts to translate the concept of cochlear nerve stimulation were not only unsuccessful, but dangerous.[1-3] Nonetheless, as computer and hearing aid technology evolved,[4] the components necessary to produce the hardware for a cochlear implant developed into what we are familiar with today. The technology that goes into the hardware was only part of the necessary considerations for CI design. Manufacturers needed to ensure biocompatibility, particularly owing to concerns of meningitis in the setting of a foreign body in a space that potentially communicates with the cerebrospinal fluid. These considerations in design for the CI were challenging and took a significant amount of time to perfect; however, the effort in perfecting the design was worthwhile, because CI became the prototype upon which many of the current electrical cranial nerve stimulators are designed.[5]

The external component consists of a microphone and a speech processor, and the internal component consists of a receiver/stimulator and electrode array. The 2 components contain a magnet that allows communication and integration of external signal to be delivered to the cochlear nerve. The microphone detects the sounds produced by the external environment and the processor converts these inputs into electrically encoded signals. Both components are worn behind the ear in current CI models. The encoded signal produced by the external components are transmitted

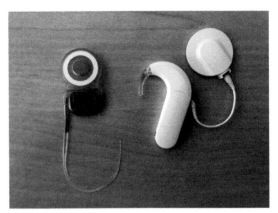

Fig. 1. Internal (*left*) and external (*right*) components of a CI. The internal receiver/stimulator shown here has a straight electrode. These components communicate through the skin and soft tissues via a magnet that connects the pieces and permits sound to be transmitted to the receiver stimulator.

to the internal receiver stimulator across the skin and soft tissues. The transmitted signal continues to the electrode arrays that sits within the scala tympani (ST) of the cochlea and send electrical stimuli to the cochlear nerve fibers. Importantly, the electrode arrays are probably the component of CI that have evolved more than any over the years (**Table 1**). The integrity and resolution of the signal introduced to the cochlear nerve is theoretically enhanced as the number of electrodes is increased.[6] Additionally, the electrode stiffness and flexibility can be altered to optimize insertion length and atraumatic insertion based on individual needs.

Relative to many of the other electrical implantable devices, the range of electrical inputs delivered by the CI is broad and complex. The CI attempts to translate environmental signals that have complex and specific spatial and temporal information and, despite significant advances in technologies, modern engineering is far from achieving restoration of natural hearing. Nonetheless, the technology and hardware that comprise the CI have been applied to various implantable stimulation devices that are used in otolaryngology (ie, hypoglossal nerve stimulator, vestibular implant, vagal

Table 1
CI electrode design overview for anatomically normal cochleae

	Standard Length	Hybrid/Electroacoustical Stimulation
Cochlear Corporation	Contour Advance: cochleostomy insertion, precurved perimodiolar electrode, 22 electrodes, 14.5–15.0 mm active length Slim Modiolar: RW or cochleostomy insertion, precurved electrode, 22 electrodes, 14.5 mm active length Slim Straight: RW or cochleostomy insertion, straight electrode, 22 electrodes, 19.1 mm active length	Hybrid L24: RW or cochleostomy insertion, straight electrode, 22 electrodes, 16 mm active length
Med-El	FLEX Series[a]: RW or cochleostomy insertion, straight electrode, 19 electrodes, various lengths 20.0–31.5 mm Classic Series: RW or cochleostomy insertion, straight electrode, 24 electrodes, various lengths 15.0–31.5 mm	FLEX Series[a]: RW insertion, straight electrode, 19 electrodes, various lengths 20.0–31.5 mm
Advanced Bionics	HiFocus Mid Scalar: RW or cochleostomy insertion, precurved mid-scalar electrode, 16 electrodes, 15 mm active length HiFocus Helix: cochleostomy insertion, precurved electrode, 16 electrodes, 13 mm active length HiFocus 1J: Cochleostomy insertion, straight electrode, 16 electrodes, 17 mm active length	HiFocus SlimJ: RW or cochleostomy insertion, straight electrode, 16 electrodes, 20 mm active length

Abbreviation: RW, round window membrane.

This table represents some of the more common electrodes and variations of electrodes used in anatomically normal cochleae. For additional, more specific electrode information, please visit each manufacturer's website.

[a] Med-El FLEX series has a variety of electrodes named based on the length of their electrode (eg, FLEX20, FLEX24, FLEX28, and FLEXSOFT [31.5 mm]) and is used in hearing preservation CI.

nerve stimulator) and have permitted restoration of sensory and functional input for a variety of otolaryngologic disorders. The following sections demonstrate how otolaryngologists have integrated CI into management of SNHL as the first cranial nerve stimulator and describe the workup and indications, surgical considerations, and outcomes in adult and pediatric CI.

PATIENT EVALUATION

The workup for CI is extensive and requires a significant amount of coordination between otolaryngologists and audiologists. Audiologic evaluation is typically the first step in the workup. This is followed by a physician evaluation, CI candidacy evaluation, and imaging before CI surgery and rehabilitation occur. We focus this discussion on audiologic evaluations, review briefly the current indications and relative contraindications for CI in adults and children, and end with a discussion on imaging as part of the workup in CI.

Audiologic Assessment

Adults
The audiologic assessment in adults can occur over the time course of many years. Most patients with postlingual deafness present with progressive bilateral SNHL, and as such, they often have multiple audiograms before being evaluated for CI candidacy. Because of the long duration of this process, many adults undergoing a CI workup have had adequate trials of hearing amplification before considering CI. Comprehensive audiometric evaluation with air and bone conduction thresholds between 250 and 8000 Hz is essential in the initial evaluations along with speech discrimination scores. Recent attention to residual low frequency hearing has made testing of 125 Hz important during the audiometric evaluation.

After comprehensive audiometry, CI candidacy testing is necessary. This is a more involved assessment that evaluates open set speech recognition score. There are a variety tests available to evaluate open set speech recognition; however, a minimum speech test battery was developed in 1996 by the American Academy of Otolaryngology–Head and Neck Surgery and the American Academy of Audiology[7] and revised in 2011.[8] Currently, adult speech recognition testing requires consonant nucleus consonant word testing and AzBio sentence testing.[9] Typically this is performed in quiet and +10 or +5 signal-to-noise ratios in a patients best aided condition. One of the challenges with interpretation of the assessment is that the neither the US Food and Drug Administration nor Centers for Medicare & Medicaid Services have not standardized a testing protocol. This lack leaves open the possibility for some variability in CI candidacy testing. Nonetheless, audiometric assessment before CI in adults is a process that begins with comprehensive audiometry and commences with open set speech recognition testing. Indications and criteria for CI are based on scores within the audiologic evaluation and discussed elsewhere in this article.

Pediatric patients
The audiologic assessment of the pediatric population is complicated by the fact that determining the degree of hearing loss in infants and children can be challenging and speech recognition testing is often not possible. After failed newborn hearing screen, the evaluation typically begins with behavioral audiometry. After an initial diagnosis of hearing loss with behavioral audiometry, an early hearing aid trial is necessary. Further physiologic confirmation of hearing loss is necessary with auditory brainstem response and otoacoustic emission. Failure to make progress with auditory and language skills despite an adequate hearing aid trial after intervention with speech

pathologists is essential for infants and children to meet CI criteria, and these interventions are paramount in the workup of the pediatric patient.

In addition to not developing age-appropriate language skills, infants and children must also have severe to profound SNHL. This is largely due to the concern of implanting a patient who may have some degree of auditory function. In infants, the audiometric workup is complete at this point, and CI can be considered. In children more than 2 years old, the lexical neighborhood test and multisyllabic lexical neighborhood test were developed as ways to evaluate speech recognition,[10] and they were added to the workup for determining CI candidacy for this age group.

The nuances and complexities of the pediatric audiologic evaluation cannot be overstated, and the workup presented here is merely on overview of the process. The challenges in evaluating a young child and making the diagnosis of hearing loss highlight the importance of a dedicated team of audiologists and speech pathologists who specialize in managing pediatric patients. As experience with the workup of pediatric patients grows, so too does the ability to feel confident with the diagnosis and intervention. There is substantial evidence that early CI improves outcomes,[11,12] and this has opened the door to offer CI for infants less than 12 months old.[13] As experience continues to evolve, it is likely that the workup and pediatric evaluation will as well.

Criteria for implantation

The indications for CI have expanded substantially in the last decade. US Food and Drug Administration indications vary slightly based on the device being implanted; however, the early indications for CI was initially reserved for postlingually deafened adult patients with severe to profound SNHL. Indications were first expanded to include prelingually deafened children more than 2 years of age around 1990, and children 12 months or older in 2000.[14] Over the ensuing decades, electrode design and surgical techniques have evolved such that hearing preservation is now possible, and there is significant early evidence to suggest benefit from combined electrical input from CI and natural, low frequency hearing.

As discussed elsewhere in this article, current indications for adult CI are based largely on understanding of open set speech, and the criteria for implantation are determined by scores of open set speech recognition (eg, AzBio, consonant nucleus consonant). Typically, scores of less than 50% on testing (40% for Centers for Medicare & Medicaid Services) is necessary for patients to meet CI candidacy. These score requirements are complex, and vary slightly for each CI Company based on US Food and Drug Administration criteria. Additionally, Medicare has a different set of criteria for patients to meet CI candidacy (**Table 2**). For the pediatric population, criteria are based on audiometric assessments and failure to develop age-appropriate language skills.

Although the list of indications is expanding, the contraindications for CI are becoming clearer as experience grows. First, patients need a cochlear nerve to undergo CI. MRI is used to determine the presence of a cochlear nerve in congenitally deaf children. Although definitive absence of a nerve is not always easy to determine, imaging that suggests the absence of a cochlear nerve or cochlear nerve dysplasia is a relative contraindication for CI, and patients who receive CI in this setting do not perform as well.[15,16] In addition, it is well-recognized that the duration of deafness is the most important factor in determining CI performance, thus prelingually deafened adult patients who have not developed language is a relative contraindication. Finally, patients who do not have the capacity or social support to undertake the rehabilitation process, should not receive CI.

Table 2
Overview of CI indications

	US Food and Drug Administration*	Medicare
Adults		
Cochlear Corporation	Moderate to profound bilateral SNHL; ≤50% on sentence recognition testing on implanted ear, <60% on contralateral ear	Moderate to profound bilateral SNHL 40% on sentence recognition testing
Med-El	Severe to profound bilateral SNHL; ≤40% on open-set sentence recognition testing in best aided condition	
Advanced Bionics	Severe to profound bilateral SNHL; ≤50% on sentence recognition testing in best aided condition	
Hearing preservation/EAS		
Cochlear Corporation	EAS: Residual low-frequency hearing, and severe to profound SNHL; aided CNC word scores between 10%–60% in ear to be implanted, ≤80% CNC in contralateral ear but not better than implanted ear	Normal to moderate hearing loss in low frequencies and severe to profound SNHL in mid to high frequencies; moderately severe to profound mid to high frequency loss in contralateral ear; aided CNC word scores ≥10% and ≤60% in ear to be implanted; ≤80% CNC in contralateral ear
Med-El	EAS: Residual low-frequency hearing, and severe to profound SNHL; aided CNC word scores ≤60% in ear to be implanted; worse thresholds and CNC scores in contralateral ear	Normal to moderate SNHL in low frequencies and severe to profound loss in mid to high frequencies; Aided CNC word scores ≤60% in ear to be implanted and contralateral ear
Pediatrics	12–24 mo: profound SNHL and limited benefit from binaural hearing aid trial 24 months–17 years: Severe to profound SNHL and limited benefit from binaural hearing aid trial; MLNT; LNT scores ≤30%	–

Limited benefits from hearing aids or binaural amplification is necessary to meet CI candidacy. Additional manufacturer- and US Food and Drug Administration-specific information can be obtained by visiting each manufacturer's website. Medicare and pediatric indications do not have manufacturer-specific indications.

Abbreviations: CNC, consonant nucleus consonant; EAS, electroacoustical stimulation; LNT, lexical neighborhood test; MLNT, multiple lexical neighborhood test.

It is interesting to note some of the challenging decision making that is required as indications are expanding. As more adult patients with natural low frequency hearing meet CI candidacy, the discussion of which ear should receive implantation requires more consideration. Despite evidence for the potential to preserve low frequency hearing, CI surgery also risks insult to the residual hearing, and the durability of hearing preservation remains unclear.[17,18] In children, this decision is often not as relevant, although the decision to perform bilateral CI in a single or sequential procedures has become relevant in this population. Certainly, evidence supports benefit from bilateral CI in children; however, it remains unclear if a single procedure offers overall benefit compared with sequential procedures.[19,20] Ultimately, as the criteria for CI evolve, the decision-making process becomes more complex, which requires comprehensive discussions among patients, family, physicians, and audiologists.

Imaging

After audiometric evaluation and determination of CI candidacy, imaging is typically necessary to evaluate inner ear structures. There is no consensus as to which imaging modality is most appropriate.[21] In the pediatric population, there is concern about exposure to radiation with computed tomography (CT) scans, and MRI is generally advocated initially.[22] The advantages of MRI in the pediatric population is that the cochlear nerve can be clearly identified on T2 sequences, and abnormalities detected on MRI may preclude CI surgery.[23] Recently, concern has been raised about the role of gadolinium-based contrast in MRI owing to controversy over deposition in the brain.[24] Thus, many newer protocols in the workup of pediatric SNHL do not require gadolinium.

In the adult population with postlingual deafness, CT scanning has been advocated if there is concern for chronic otitis media or a history of middle ear disease, whereas MRI would be favored with a history of meningitis or asymmetrical SNHL.[25,26] Irrespective of the imaging modality chosen, visualization of the cochlea is essential before CI. Although imaging often has little influence on the approach to CI surgery in postlingually deafened adults, it provides necessary insights in the evaluation of pediatric SNHL that can have a major impact of CI decision making.

COCHLEAR IMPLANT SURGERY

A comprehensive review of surgical techniques in CI is outside the scope of this article. Nonetheless, we introduce the basic techniques used in CI surgery. Before introducing these techniques, there are 2 special considerations that warrant mentioning in CI surgery. First, in the modern day of CI surgery, facial nerve monitoring is routinely used in almost all otologic and neurotologic procedures that require mastoidectomy.[27] Thus, it should be communicated with the anesthesiologist that paralytic agents should be avoided during the induction of anesthesia. In CI surgery, 2-channel electrodes that monitor upper and lower divisions of the facial nerve suffice. The second consideration during CI, monopolar electrocautery should be avoided after the implant enters the surgical field. This factor is relevant for patients undergoing bilateral CI or receiving their second-side CI. Although that cadaveric studies[28] and case reports[29] have not demonstrated any damage to the patient or the implant itself, there is concern and risk of inducing electrical current through the electrode of the CI with monopolar cautery. Owing to this risk, monopolar cautery should not be used routinely in patients with an existing CI.

Techniques

Although a variety of techniques have been described for CI, the classical approach is a facial recess/posterior tympanotomy approach that is used in both children and adults.[30] It allows access to the round window membrane and cochlear promontory with a relatively direct route for electrode insertion with few serious complications.[31] Fixation techniques for the device have become more minimalistic as the tight pocket techniques become more familiar.[32] This more minimalistic approach also decreased the likelihood of rare, but potentially devastating intracranial complications encountered with the drilling of a well for fixation.[33]

Additional alternative techniques have been described, but are largely reserved for patients with anatomic variations that call for deviation from the facial recess approach.[34] The most well-described alternative approach is the suprameatal approach.[35] This approach requires a tympanomeatal flap to be raised for access to the round window; however, it avoids the need to drill a facial recess, and thus decreases risk to the facial nerve.[36] Rarely used techniques such as a middle fossa and canal wall down approaches have been described for CI, but are not considered for routine use.[37,38]

Irrespective of the surgical approach, the goal is to place the CI electrode within the ST (**Fig. 2**). Placement within the ST optimizes the interaction between the electrode and the spiral ganglion cells, which are being directly stimulated. It has been well-demonstrated that user outcomes are improved with the electrodes in the ST,[39,40] and any translocation to the scala vestibuli decreases performance. Although cochleostomy was traditionally used to gain access to the ST, round window and extended round window approaches have gained popularity owing to the increased likelihood of ST placement.[40,41] Additionally, as soft surgery techniques become standard, round window membrane insertions have been favored because they avoid the potential trauma of drilling a cochleostomy.[42]

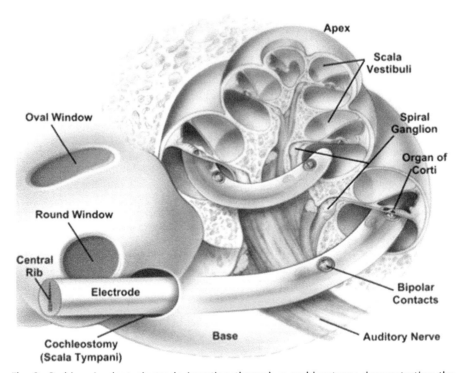

Fig. 2. Cochlear implant electrode insertion through a cochleostomy demonstrating the optimal course through the ST. Insertion into the ST optimizes transmission of stimuli to the spiral ganglion neurons. (*From* Zeng FG, Popper AN, Fay RR, editors. Auditory prostheses: Cochlear implants and beyond. New York (NY): Springer-Verlag; 2004; with permission.)

Special Considerations in Surgery

The techniques described in this article can be used for routine CI in children and adults with normal cochlear anatomy. Nonetheless, there are certain situations that warrant special consideration during CI surgery. We will focus on a few of these situations described here.

Children Less Than 12 Months Old

Although CI in children is performed with similar techniques as described for adults, certain modifications should be considered when operating on young children less than 12 months of age. The first consideration is that children this young have thinner skulls and significantly smaller mastoid cavities. Despite this smaller anatomy, the cochlear structures are fully developed in utero; thus, electrode insertion is typically achieved in cochleae without fibrosis or obstruction. Additionally, their circulating volume is significantly smaller than older children and adults, so efficient hemostasis is necessary to prevent excessive blood loss, because even small volume loss can cause circulatory concerns. This necessitates efficiency in the operating room to avoid anesthetic time. It should also be noted that their mastoid cavities often have a higher content of marrow that tends to bleed more, but can be managed with diamond burrs and bone wax typically. A final consideration in this group is that their facial nerve often courses laterally as it exists the mastoid at the stylomastoid foramen. This variation requires more careful planning of the postauricular incision and avoidance of deeper dissections at the mastoid tip. Similarly, care to avoid aggressive raising of the periosteum inferiorly is necessary to prevent traction injury on the laterally placed nerve. Despite all the things to consider intraoperatively in young children, CI surgical outcomes have generally mirrored those of children greater than 12 months old.[43,44]

Cochlear Malformation

Radiographically detectable cochleovestibular malformations are thought to be present in roughly 20% to 30% of patients with congenital hearing loss.[45] Jackler and associates[46] described the earliest classification based on organogenesis and radiographic abnormalities; however, newer classification systems have been developed that divide anomalies into parts I and II incomplete partition anomalies.[47] Experience has taught the CI surgeon that challenges should be expected during implantation of the malformed cochlea. This situation makes preoperative imaging essential in the evaluation of children with congenital hearing loss who are considering CI. There is lack of consensus on the preferred imaging modality, and both CT scans and MRIs are useful.[45] Intraoperatively, facial nerve anomalies and cerebrospinal fluid leak should also be expected, because they often accompany cochlear malformations and can complicate CI surgery.[48]

It is beyond the scope of this article to describe all the cochleovestibular anomalies; nonetheless, it is relevant to describe how some of the anomalies influence CI surgical decision making. Many of the anomalies, such as partition anomalies and enlarged vestibular aqueducts, have relatively normal cochlear anatomy. Although these subtle abnormalities may introduce the risk of a cerebrospinal fluid gusher,[49] electrode choice and surgical technique is unlikely to be influenced by the more subtle anomalies. Anomalies with more significant abnormalities such as common cavity require more caution during electrode insertion as inadvertent insertion into the IAC or carotid canal has been described and the rate of facial stimulation is elevated.[50]

Owing to the variety of cochleovestibular anomalies, outcomes with CI can vary irrespective of technique or electrode. Milder abnormalities such as incomplete partition anomalies and enlarged vestibular aqueduct can perform well with CI,[51,52] whereas more severe abnormalities such as common cavity are less likely to achieve significant speech development.[53,54]

Cochlear Ossificans (Labyrinthitis Ossificans)

There are few scenarios where the cochlea can be obstructed with ossified tissues that make electrode insertion challenging. Often cochlear ossification occurs secondary to meningitis, although far-advanced otosclerosis can induce a similar process.[55,56] In this setting, efficient workup and surgical scheduling is necessary because ossification can progress rapidly and limit electrode insertion.

Ossification after bacterial meningitis presumably occurs after the spread of infection to the cochlea through the cochlear aqueduct.[57] The inflammatory reaction within the cochlea progresses through various phases that starts as fibrosis and culminates with ossification that has its most dramatic effect at basal turn of the cochlea, although the entire cochlea can be affected.[58] In the setting of advanced otosclerosis, ossification typically occurs at the round window and extends to the basal turn of the cochlea.[59] In the majority of cases, ossification does not extend beyond the basal turn of the cochlea. To overcome the ossification that is encountered, various drill out techniques have been described that can be performed with the standard posterior tympanotomy approach.[60,61] If access for drill out of the ossified portion of the cochlea is limited, canal wall down and cavity obliteration has been described.[62] Additionally, other techniques that describe scala vestibuli insertion[63,64] and retrograde electrode insertion have been described.[65]

Surgically, not only is insertion challenging, ossification in the setting of meningitis and otosclerosis has higher reported rates of facial nerve stimulation that in traditional CI.[59,66] There is also evidence demonstrating that patients with cochlear ossificans who undergo CI often have limited audiometric benefit,[67,68] which may be because the spiral ganglion neurons can be affected by the ossification process.[58,69]

Hearing Preservation Surgery

As the indications for CI have expanded to include patients with residual low-frequency hearing, the surgical approach in those candidates has evolved. Soft surgery techniques are essential in these candidates because avoiding trauma is necessary to preserve their remaining natural hearing.[70] In addition to these surgical techniques, some have advocated for oral steroids in the perioperative period with the administration of topical corticosteroids before electrode insertion.[71,72] There is a preponderance of evidence to suggest that the combination of electric and acoustical hearing offers benefit beyond what CI alone can offer.[73–76] Collectively, the term for this is electroacoustic stimulation. Given that the residual hearing is available in the low frequencies, shorter electrodes have been designed to avoid potential damage to the remaining apical hair cells. Although there is the theoretic concern about lack of input to that region as the process of hair cell degeneration continues, auditory outcomes have demonstrated stability with the shorter electrode arrays.[77] As our ability to understand the factors that impact hearing preservation improve, the outcomes should continue to improve. However, this approach to CI remains relatively new, and more research evaluating these long-term results is necessary.

OUTCOMES

The evolution of CI technology, indications, and techniques has created an evolution in our evaluation of outcomes. Within our specialty, otolaryngologists have set higher expectations with CI as experience is gained. Many of the current outcomes and expectations for CI users are not similar to the expectations for CI users of the early generations. For example, many appropriate prelingually deaf pediatric CI candidates can reasonably expect to attain speech development that supersedes that of prelingually deafened children who do not undergo CI.[12] Although the literature varies somewhat in its assessment of speech outcomes in pediatric CI, the consistent finding in this research has been that earlier access to auditory input with CI improves a child's acquisition of language.[78,79] Many pediatric CI patients are able to enter mainstream education systems[80,81]; however, challenges in this setting are documented.[82] These achievements in children who receive CI are now considered the expectation. Similar to the pediatric population, postlingually deafened adult CI candidates can expect reasonable open set speech recognition within a few months after implantation.[83] Not only is open set speech improved in CI users, music appreciation can be obtained with the appropriate training.[84,85]

Despite these expectations and good outcomes for a majority of CI recipients, there is a significant amount that is not understood about what affects outcomes in CI. The important factors that influence CI performance have not changed significantly over time, and age at implantation and duration of deafness continue to be the most important factors.[86] Newer research is looking at details of electrode location within the cochlea as a factor that can have a significant impact of CI performance.[87] Intraoperative CT scans[88] and electrocochleography can also be used to aid the surgeon in atraumatic electrode placement, and may play a role in improving outcomes.[89] It remains to be seen how these new factors will influence patient outcomes, yet these advances are likely to continue to motivate otolaryngologists to reach new expectations that will likely continue the trend of positive patient outcomes.

FUTURE CONSIDERATIONS

There has been significant change in the engineering and technology of CI over the past decades. What started as a single channel cochlear nerve stimulator that was incompatible with MRI has evolved into a multiple channel, atraumatic, MRI-compatible cochlear nerve stimulator. Some of the newer technologies even allow CI to measure electrical potentials during CI insertion.[90,91] Despite these changes, the concepts behind the CI as a cranial nerve stimulator have remained constant. It is possible that the future of CI will represent a paradigm shift in the way in which neural stimulation occurs. Significant research is exploring more complex techniques for cochlear nerve stimulation that involve piezoelectric stimulators,[92,93] totally implantable stimulators,[94] and optogenetic[95,96] mechanisms of neural stimulation. The goal underlying these various novel techniques is to improve the integrity of the signal being delivered to the cochlear nerve. As this work becomes more refined, the future for CI seems to be limitless in its capacity to restore auditory input to deaf patients, and the potential changes of the upcoming years holds significant promise. If the future decades are anything like the decades that preceded it, CI will continue to be a revolutionary medical device.

REFERENCES

1. Eisen MD. Djourno, Eyries, and the first implanted electrical neural stimulator to restore hearing. Otol Neurotol 2003;24:500–6.

2. Shah SB, Chung JH, Jackler RK. Lodestones, quackery, and science: electrical stimulation of the ear before cochlear implants. Am J Otol 1997;18:665–70.

3. Mudry A, Mills M. The early history of the cochlear implant: a retrospective. JAMA Otolaryngol Head Neck Surg 2013;139:446–53.

4. Mills M. Hearing aids and the history of electronics miniaturization. IEEE Ann Hist Comput 2011;33(2):24–44.

5. Eisele DW, Schwartz AR, Smith PL. Tongue neuromuscular and direct hypoglossal nerve stimulation for obstructive sleep apnea. Otolaryngol Clin North Am 2003;36:501–10.

6. Clark G. The multi-channel cochlear implant: past, present and future perspectives. Cochlear Implants Int 2009;10(Suppl 1):2–13.

7. Nilsson MJ, McCaw VM, Soli S. Minimum Speech Test Battery for Adult Cochlear Implant Users. Los Angeles: House Ear Institute; 1996.

8. MSTB. Minimum speech test battery for adult cochlear implant users. Available at: http://wwwauditorypotentialcom/MSTBfiles/MSTBManual2011-06-20%20pdf 2011. Accessed April 9, 2019.

9. Spahr AJ, Dorman MF, Litvak LM, et al. Development and validation of the AzBio sentence lists. Ear Hear 2012;33:112–7.

10. Kirk KI, Pisoni DB, Osberger MJ. Lexical effects on spoken word recognition by pediatric cochlear implant users. Ear Hear 1995;16:470–81.

11. Yoshinaga-Itano C, Sedey AL, Wiggin M, et al. Language outcomes improved through early hearing detection and earlier cochlear implantation. Otol Neurotol 2018;39:1256–63.

12. Niparko JK, Tobey EA, Thal DJ, et al. Spoken language development in children following cochlear implantation. JAMA 2010;303:1498–506.

13. Holman MA, Carlson ML, Driscoll CL, et al. Cochlear implantation in children 12 months of age and younger. Otol Neurotol 2013;34:251–8.

14. Cochlear Implants. 2010. Available at: https://report.nih.gov/nihfactsheets/ViewFactSheet.aspx?csid=83. Accessed April 1, 2019.

15. Peng KA, Kuan EC, Hagan S, et al. Cochlear nerve aplasia and hypoplasia: predictors of cochlear implant success. Otolaryngol Head Neck Surg 2017;157:392–400.

16. Birman CS, Powell HR, Gibson WP, et al. Cochlear implant outcomes in cochlea nerve aplasia and hypoplasia. Otol Neurotol 2016;37:438–45.

17. Moteki H, Nishio SY, Miyagawa M, et al. Long-term results of hearing preservation cochlear implant surgery in patients with residual low frequency hearing. Acta Otolaryngol 2017;137:516–21.

18. Brant JA, Ruckenstein MJ. Electrode selection for hearing preservation in cochlear implantation: a review of the evidence. World J Otorhinolaryngol Head Neck Surg 2016;2:157–60.

19. Bianchin G, Tribi L, Formigoni P, et al. Sequential pediatric bilateral cochlear implantation: the effect of time interval between implants. Int J Pediatr Otorhinolaryngol 2017;102:10–4.

20. Uecker FC, Szczepek A, Olze H. Pediatric bilateral cochlear implantation: simultaneous versus sequential surgery. Otol Neurotol 2019;40:e454–60.

21. Tamplen M, Schwalje A, Lustig L, et al. Utility of preoperative computed tomography and magnetic resonance imaging in adult and pediatric cochlear implant candidates. Laryngoscope 2016;126:1440–5.

22. Siu JM, Blaser SI, Gordon KA, et al. Efficacy of a selective imaging paradigm prior to pediatric cochlear implantation. Laryngoscope 2019. [Epub ahead of print].

23. Parry DA, Booth T, Roland PS. Advantages of magnetic resonance imaging over computed tomography in preoperative evaluation of pediatric cochlear implant candidates. Otol Neurotol 2005;26:976–82.

24. Pullicino R, Radon M, Biswas S, et al. A review of the current evidence on gadolinium deposition in the brain. Clin Neuroradiol 2018;28:159–69.

25. Jiang ZY, Odiase E, Isaacson B, et al. Utility of MRIs in adult cochlear implant evaluations. Otol Neurotol 2014;35:1533–5.

26. Mackeith S, Joy R, Robinson P, et al. Pre-operative imaging for cochlear implantation: magnetic resonance imaging, computed tomography, or both? Cochlear Implants Int 2012;13:133–6.

27. Hsieh HS, Wu CM, Zhuo MY, et al. Intraoperative facial nerve monitoring during cochlear implant surgery: an observational study. Medicine (Baltimore) 2015; 94:e456.

28. Jeyakumar A, Wilson M, Sorrel JE, et al. Monopolar cautery and adverse effects on cochlear implants. JAMA Otolaryngol Head Neck Surg 2013;139:694–7.

29. Tien DA, Woodson EA, Anne S. Safety of monopolar electrocautery in patients with cochlear implants. Ann Otol Rhinol Laryngol 2016;125:701–3.

30. Clark GM, Pyman BC, Bailey QR. The surgery for multiple-electrode cochlear implantations. J Laryngol Otol 1979;93:215–23.

31. Farinetti A, Ben Gharbia D, Mancini J, et al. Cochlear implant complications in 403 patients: comparative study of adults and children and review of the literature. Eur Ann Otorhinolaryngol Head Neck Dis 2014;131:177–82.

32. Balkany TJ, Whitley M, Shapira Y, et al. The temporalis pocket technique for cochlear implantation: an anatomic and clinical study. Otol Neurotol 2009;30: 903–7.

33. Gosepath J, Maurer J, Mann WJ. Epidural hematoma after cochlear implantation in a 2.5-year-old boy. Otol Neurotol 2005;26:202–4.

34. Surmelioglu O, Ozdemir S, Tarkan O, et al. Alternative techniques in cochlear implantation. J Int Adv Otol 2016;12:109–12.

35. Kronenberg J, Migirov L, Dagan T. Suprameatal approach: new surgical approach for cochlear implantation. J Laryngol Otol 2001;115:283–5.

36. Postelmans JT, Tange RA, Stokroos RJ, et al. The suprameatal approach: a safe alternative surgical technique for cochlear implantation. Otol Neurotol 2010;31: 196–203.

37. Carfrae MJ, Foyt D. Intact meatal skin, canal wall down approach for difficult cochlear implantation. J Laryngol Otol 2009;123:903–6.

38. Bittencourt AG, Tsuji RK, Tempestini JP, et al. Cochlear implantation through the middle cranial fossa: a novel approach to access the basal turn of the cochlea. Braz J Otorhinolaryngol 2013;79:158–62.

39. Wanna GB, Noble JH, McRackan TR, et al. Assessment of electrode placement and audiological outcomes in bilateral cochlear implantation. Otol Neurotol 2011; 32:428–32.

40. O'Connell BP, Cakir A, Hunter JB, et al. Electrode location and angular insertion depth are predictors of audiologic outcomes in cochlear implantation. Otol Neurotol 2016;37:1016–23.

41. Roland PS, Wright CG, Isaacson B. Cochlear implant electrode insertion: the round window revisited. Laryngoscope 2007;117:1397–402.

42. Yu H, Tong B, Zhang Q, et al. Drill-induced noise level during cochleostomy. Acta Otolaryngol 2014;134:943–6.

43. James AL, Papsin BC. Cochlear implant surgery at 12 months of age or younger. Laryngoscope 2004;114:2191–5.

44. Roland JT Jr, Cosetti M, Wang KH, et al. Cochlear implantation in the very young child: long-term safety and efficacy. Laryngoscope 2009;119:2205–10.
45. Huang BY, Zdanski C, Castillo M. Pediatric sensorineural hearing loss, part 1: practical aspects for neuroradiologists. AJNR Am J Neuroradiol 2012;33:211–7.
46. Jackler RK, Luxford WM, House WF. Congenital malformations of the inner ear: a classification based on embryogenesis. Laryngoscope 1987;97:2–14.
47. Sennaroglu L, Saatci I. A new classification for cochleovestibular malformations. Laryngoscope 2002;112:2230–41.
48. Papsin BC. Cochlear implantation in children with anomalous cochleovestibular anatomy. Laryngoscope 2005;115:1–26.
49. Pakdaman MN, Herrmann BS, Curtin HD, et al. Cochlear implantation in children with anomalous cochleovestibular anatomy: a systematic review. Otolaryngol Head Neck Surg 2012;146:180–90.
50. Bloom JD, Rizzi MD, Germiller JA. Real-time intraoperative computed tomography to assist cochlear implant placement in the malformed inner ear. Otol Neurotol 2009;30:23–6.
51. Manzoor NF, Wick CC, Wahba M, et al. Bilateral sequential cochlear implantation in patients with enlarged vestibular aqueduct (EVA) syndrome. Otol Neurotol 2016;37:e96–103.
52. Farhood Z, Nguyen SA, Miller SC, et al. Cochlear implantation in inner ear malformations: systematic review of speech perception outcomes and intraoperative findings. Otolaryngol Head Neck Surg 2017;156:783–93.
53. Pradhananga RB, Thomas JK, Natarajan K, et al. Long term outcome of cochlear implantation in five children with common cavity deformity. Int J Pediatr Otorhinolaryngol 2015;79:685–9.
54. Zhang L, Qiu J, Qin F, et al. Cochlear implantation outcomes in children with common cavity deformity; a retrospective study. J Otol 2017;12:138–42.
55. Green JD Jr, Marion MS, Hinojosa R. Labyrinthitis ossificans: histopathologic consideration for cochlear implantation. Otolaryngol Head Neck Surg 1991;104:320–6.
56. Vashishth A, Fulcheri A, Prasad SC, et al. Cochlear implantation in cochlear ossification: retrospective review of etiologies, surgical considerations, and auditory outcomes. Otol Neurotol 2018;39:17–28.
57. Tinling SP, Colton J, Brodie HA. Location and timing of initial osteoid deposition in postmeningitic labyrinthitis ossificans determined by multiple fluorescent labels. Laryngoscope 2004;114:675–80.
58. Kaya S, Paparella MM, Cureoglu S. Pathologic findings of the cochlea in labyrinthitis ossificans associated with the round window membrane. Otolaryngol Head Neck Surg 2016;155:635–40.
59. Vashishth A, Fulcheri A, Rossi G, et al. Cochlear implantation in otosclerosis: surgical and auditory outcomes with a brief on facial nerve stimulation. Otol Neurotol 2017;38:e345–53.
60. Balkany T, Luntz M, Telischi FF, et al. Intact canal wall drill-out procedure for implantation of the totally ossified cochlea. Am J Otol 1997;18:S58–9.
61. Balkany T, Bird PA, Hodges AV, et al. Surgical technique for implantation of the totally ossified cochlea. Laryngoscope 1998;108:988–92.
62. Gantz BJ, McCabe BF, Tyler RS. Use of multichannel cochlear implants in obstructed and obliterated cochleas. Otolaryngol Head Neck Surg 1988;98:72–81.
63. Trudel M, Cote M, Philippon D, et al. Comparative impacts of scala vestibuli versus scala tympani cochlear implantation on auditory performances and

programming parameters in partially ossified cochleae. Otol Neurotol 2018;39: 700–6.

64. Berrettini S, Forli F, Neri E, et al. Scala vestibuli cochlear implantation in patients with partially ossified cochleas. J Laryngol Otol 2002;116:946–50.

65. Senn P, Rostetter C, Arnold A, et al. Retrograde cochlear implantation in postmeningitic basal turn ossification. Laryngoscope 2012;122:2043–50.

66. Nassiri AM, Yawn RJ, Dedmon MM, et al. Facial nerve stimulation patterns associated with cochlear implantation in labyrinthitis ossificans. Otol Neurotol 2018; 39:e992–5.

67. Rauch SD, Herrmann BS, Davis LA, et al. Nucleus 22 cochlear implantation results in postmeningitic deafness. Laryngoscope 1997;107:1606–9.

68. Liu CC, Sweeney M, Booth TN, et al. The impact of postmeningitic labyrinthitis ossificans on speech performance after pediatric cochlear implantation. Otol Neurotol 2015;36:1633–7.

69. Hinojosa R, Green JD Jr, Marion MS. Ganglion cell populations in labyrinthitis ossificans. Am J Otol 1991;12(Suppl):3–7 [discussion: 18–21].

70. Friedland DR, Runge-Samuelson C. Soft cochlear implantation: rationale for the surgical approach. Trends Amplif 2009;13:124–38.

71. Sweeney AD, Carlson ML, Zuniga MG, et al. Impact of perioperative oral steroid use on low-frequency hearing preservation after cochlear implantation. Otol Neurotol 2015;36:1480–5.

72. Cho HS, Lee KY, Choi H, et al. Dexamethasone is one of the factors minimizing the inner ear damage from electrode insertion in cochlear implantation. Audiol Neurootol 2016;21:178–86.

73. Gifford RH, Dorman MF, Skarzynski H, et al. Cochlear implantation with hearing preservation yields significant benefit for speech recognition in complex listening environments. Ear Hear 2013;34:413–25.

74. Sato M, Baumhoff P, Tillein J, et al. Physiological mechanisms in combined electric-acoustic stimulation. Otol Neurotol 2017;38:e215–23.

75. Roland JT Jr, Gantz BJ, Waltzman SB, et al. United States multicenter clinical trial of the cochlear nucleus hybrid implant system. Laryngoscope 2016;126:175–81.

76. Roland JT Jr, Gantz BJ, Waltzman SB, et al. Long-term outcomes of cochlear implantation in patients with high-frequency hearing loss. Laryngoscope 2018;128: 1939–45.

77. Gantz BJ, Dunn CC, Oleson J, et al. Acoustic plus electric speech processing: long-term results. Laryngoscope 2018;128:473–81.

78. Geers AE, Nicholas JG, Sedey AL. Language skills of children with early cochlear implantation. Ear Hear 2003;24:46S–58S.

79. Moog JS, Geers AE. Early educational placement and later language outcomes for children with cochlear implants. Otol Neurotol 2010;31:1315–9.

80. Geers AE, Brenner CA, Tobey EA. Long-term outcomes of cochlear implantation in early childhood: sample characteristics and data collection methods. Ear Hear 2011;32:2S–12S.

81. Spencer LJ, Gantz BJ, Knutson JF. Outcomes and achievement of students who grew up with access to cochlear implants. Laryngoscope 2004;114:1576–81.

82. Fitzpatrick EM, Olds J. Practitioners' perspectives on the functioning of school-age children with cochlear implants. Cochlear Implants Int 2015;16:9–23.

83. Massa ST, Ruckenstein MJ. Comparing the performance plateau in adult cochlear implant patients using HINT and AzBio. Otol Neurotol 2014;35:598–604.

84. Gu X, Liu B, Liu Z, et al. A follow-up study on music and lexical tone perception in adult mandarin-speaking cochlear implant users. Otol Neurotol 2017;38:e421–8.

85. Jiam NT, Deroche ML, Jiradejvong P, et al. A randomized controlled crossover study of the impact of online music training on pitch and timbre perception in cochlear implant users. J Assoc Res Otolaryngol 2019;20(3):247–62.

86. Blamey P, Artieres F, Baskent D, et al. Factors affecting auditory performance of postlinguistically deaf adults using cochlear implants: an update with 2251 patients. Audiol Neurootol 2013;18:36–47.

87. Chakravorti S, Noble JH, Gifford RH, et al. Further evidence of the relationship between cochlear implant electrode positioning and hearing outcomes. Otol Neurotol 2019;40(5):617–24.

88. Yamamoto N, Okano T, Yamazaki H, et al. Intraoperative evaluation of cochlear implant electrodes using mobile cone-beam computed tomography. Otol Neurotol 2019;40:177–83.

89. McClellan JH, Formeister EJ, Merwin WH 3rd, et al. Round window electrocochleography and speech perception outcomes in adult cochlear implant subjects: comparison with audiometric and biographical information. Otol Neurotol 2014;35:e245–52.

90. Calloway NH, Fitzpatrick DC, Campbell AP, et al. Intracochlear electrocochleography during cochlear implantation. Otol Neurotol 2014;35:1451–7.

91. O'Connell BP, Holder JT, Dwyer RT, et al. Intra- and postoperative electrocochleography may be predictive of final electrode position and postoperative hearing preservation. Front Neurosci 2017;11:291.

92. Yip M, Jin R, Nakajima HH, et al. A fully-implantable cochlear implant SoC with piezoelectric middle-ear sensor and arbitrary waveform neural stimulation. IEEE J Solid-State Circuits 2015;50:214–29.

93. Mukherjee N, Roseman RD, Willging JP. The piezoelectric cochlear implant: concept, feasibility, challenges, and issues. J Biomed Mater Res 2000;53:181–7.

94. Mitchell-Innes A, Saeed SR, Irving R. The future of cochlear implant design. Adv Otorhinolaryngol 2018;81:105–13.

95. Wrobel C, Dieter A, Huet A, et al. Optogenetic stimulation of cochlear neurons activates the auditory pathway and restores auditory-driven behavior in deaf adult gerbils. Sci Transl Med 2018;10 [pii:eaao0540].

96. Moser T. Optogenetic stimulation of the auditory pathway for research and future prosthetics. Curr Opin Neurobiol 2015;34:29–36.

Auditory Brainstem Implantation

Candidacy Evaluation, Operative Technique, and Outcomes

Nicholas L. Deep, MD, J. Thomas Roland Jr, MD*

KEYWORDS

- Auditory brainstem implant • Hearing loss • Auditory prosthesis
- Electric stimulation • Auditory nerve • Neurofibromatosis type 2

KEY POINTS

- The auditory brainstem implant (ABI) is a central neural auditory prosthesis for patients with profound sensorineural hearing loss who are not cochlear implant candidates, because of absence of a cochlear nerve, cochlear aplasia, or an unimplantable (completely ossified) cochlea.
- The ABI consists of a multielectrode surface array placed over the cochlear nucleus within the lateral recess of the fourth ventricle.
- The current criteria for use in the United States are NF2 patients 12 years or older undergoing first- or second-side vestibular schwannoma removal.
- The most common indications for ABI are NF2 patients; however, there are other nontumor conditions in which patients may benefit from an ABI, including bilateral cochlear nerve avulsion from trauma, complete ossification of the cochlea because of meningitis, or a severe cochlear malformation not amendable to cochlear implantation.
- There is growing experience with ABI in infants and children with encouraging outcomes.

INTRODUCTION

Options for hearing rehabilitation are dictated by the nature and cause of the hearing loss. Although multichannel cochlear implantation (CI) is an extremely effective method of hearing rehabilitation for congenital and acquired sensorineural hearing loss, there remains a population of patients with conditions that involve the cochlea

Financial Material & Support: Internal departmental funding was used without commercial sponsorship or support.

Conflicts of Interest to Declare: J.T. Roland is a consultant for Cochlear Americas and receives research grant money.

Department of Otolaryngology–Head and Neck Surgery, New York University School of Medicine, 550 1st Avenue, New York, NY 10016, USA

* Corresponding author. 550 1st Avenue, Skirball Suite 7Q, New York, NY 10016.

E-mail address: J.Thomas.RolandJr@nyulangone.org

or cochlear nerve that make peripheral cochlear stimulation ineffective or impossible, and such patients may not receive adequate benefit from a cochlear implant. Most commonly, this situation occurs in patients with neurofibromatosis type 2 (NF2), in which bilateral vestibular schwannoma growth or surgical removal results in loss of cochlear nerve function. In this situation, direct electric stimulation of the cochlear nucleus at the brainstem using an auditory brainstem implant (ABI) is possible.

House and Hitselberger reported the first results of an ABI in 1979 after placing the ABI electrode via translabyrinthine craniotomy at the time of vestibular schwannoma removal.[1,2] The first implant was a platinum electrode pair with 0.5-mm balls separated by 1.5 mm that was placed within the brainstem in the region of the cochlear nucleus. Initially, the patient did well and reported benefit with enhanced lip reading and environmental sound awareness. Over time, however, her performance deteriorated, which was attributed to electrode migration. As a result, future iterations of device design were aimed at reducing electrode migration.

In 2000, the Food and Drug Administration approved the use of a multichannel ABI in patients 12 years of age and older diagnosed with NF2. In more recent years, particularly in Europe and countries outside of the United States, growing experience with ABIs in non-NF2 indications (bilateral total ossified cochlea, inner ear malformations, bilateral temporal bone fractures) have been reported.[3–6] Furthermore, studies to expand ABI indications to children and infants who are not cochlear implant candidates are underway. Colletti and coworkers[7] performed the first pediatric ABI surgery for auditory nerve aplasia in 2001, which established the feasibility of this device in the pediatric population.

To date, more than 1000 ABI procedures have been performed worldwide.[8] Results have been mixed, but the ABI continues to offer hope for a population of patients who otherwise do not have access to the auditory world. Although the speech perception benefits are usually modest at best, the auditory information can serve to aid with lip reading, and provide protective and quality of life benefits from hearing environmental sounds.[9,10]

AUDITORY BRAINSTEM IMPLANT DESIGN AND FUNCTION

Similar to a cochlear implant, the ABI device includes external and internal components. The external components include the microphone, battery, speech processor, external magnet, and transmitter antenna. The internal components include the internal magnet, antenna, receiver-stimulator, and an electrode array (**Fig. 1**). Sound is first detected by a microphone (worn on the ear) and converted into an electrical signal. This signal is then sent to an external sound processor where it is transformed into an electronic code. This code is transmitted via radiofrequency through the skin by a transmitting coil that is held externally over the receiver–stimulator by a magnet. Subsequently, this code is translated by the receiver–stimulator into rapid electrical impulses distributed to individual wires that travel along the array to the electrode contacts, which are housed within a soft silicone paddle that is placed along the surface of the brainstem, thereby allowing direct stimulation of the cochlear nucleus.

Because the tonotopicity of the cochlear nucleus is arranged obliquely through the pons, an ABI with penetrating electrodes has been designed to selectively stimulate frequencies that are located in areas deep to the surface. However, results, of the penetrating ABI implant have not demonstrated an advantage over surface electrodes, in part because of the difficulty in definitively identifying the cochlear nucleus before placement.[11] Midbrain implants placed on the dorsal surface of the inferior colliculus have also been reported for patients with a damaged or dysfunctional cochlear nucleus, to stimulate the auditory pathway more proximally.

A   **B**   **C**

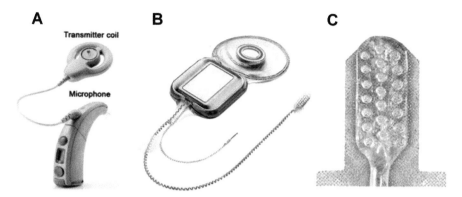

Fig. 1. Cochlear Corporation ABI device. (*A*) External component including microphone, sound processor, and magnet. (*B*) Internal component including the receiver-stimulator and electrode array. (*C*) Close-up view of the electrode contact paddle, which interfaces with the brainstem. (*Courtesy of* Cochlear Ltd, Macquarie University, Sydney, Australia; with permission.)

In the United States, the only Food and Drug Administration–approved ABI device is by Cochlear Corporation (Sydney, Australia). The latest model (ABI541) features 21 platinum electrode contacts along the paddle, which measures 8.5 × 3.0 mm and is designed to work with the Nucleus 6 sound processor (see **Fig. 1**). MED-EL Corporation (Innsbruck, Austria) and Oticon Medical (Vallauris, France) also manufacture ABI devices that are used outside of the United States.

CANDIDACY EVALUATION

Evaluation for candidacy should be performed by a multidisciplinary team involving neurotology, neurosurgery, audiology, speech therapy, and neuropsychology. An ABI is indicated for patients with bilateral profound hearing loss because of an absent or nonfunctional cochlear nerve and/or an absent or unimplantable cochlea. The most common candidates are patients with NF2 who have undergone tumor resection with known loss of their cochlear nerve. However, in nontumor patients, candidacy evaluation should first ensure that a cochlear implant is not a feasible option, because of the superior audiometric outcomes with cochlear implantation compared with ABI. An MRI of the brain is used to evaluate the patency of the cochlea and the presence or absence of the cochlear nerve. Heavily T2-weighted MRI is superior to high-resolution computed tomography for detecting subtle cochlear fibrosis. In patients without vestibular schwannoma, parasagittal thin-slice MRI through the bilateral internal auditory canals are used determine the presence and size of the cochlear nerves. Additionally, computed tomography may complement MRI by evaluating for a patent cochlear nerve aperture between the internal auditory canal and modiolus. Radiographic evidence of an absent cochlea is a straightforward indication for ABI. However, radiographic evidence of cochlear nerve aplasia is less straightforward because resolution is limited in identifying very thin cochlear nerves or those running with the facial nerve, even when using high-resolution T2-weighted MRI sequences (eg, CISS, FIESTA). Several publications have shown an occult connection between the peripheral and central auditory pathways in the presence of an otherwise absent cochlear nerve radiographically.[12–14] For these reasons, functional tests of the auditory pathway, including conventional audiometry or promontory stimulation testing, remains the gold standard for determining the presence of a cochlear nerve.[13] Patients with gross sound perception or sound perception after promontory stimulation should first undergo cochlear implantation.

There are several conditions whereby a patient with NF2 should also undergo cochlear implantation before considering ABI, including those with stable or radiated tumors and in those who have previously undergone microsurgical tumor resection with preservation of the cochlear nerve. In patients with a history of tumor removal whereby the status of the cochlear nerve is uncertain, use of promontory stimulation may be performed.[15,16] This should be done no sooner than 6 to 8 weeks after surgery to allow for neuropraxia to resolve.[17] Of note, an absent promontory stimulation waveform does not exclude the possibility that the patient will derive benefit with a cochlear implant.[16] Because cochlear implant surgery is performed on an outpatient basis and has a favorable risk profile when compared with ABI surgery, it is often attempted before ABI when feasible. If successful, a cochlear implant could provide open-set speech recognition in up to 70% of cases, which is significantly better than what is achieved with an ABI.[18,19]

In patients with NF2, obtaining an MRI before placement of an implant also provides them with their last opportunity to obtain a high-quality brain image without artifact or the need to remove a magnet. Additional MRI of the entire neuroaxis is important in patients with NF2 because the presence of tumors along the spine may result in neurologic changes during surgery or may complicate the ability to perform a lumbar puncture during the postoperative period in the event of a cerebrospinal fluid (CSF) leak or suspected meningitis.

INDICATIONS

Candidates for ABI can broadly be classified into two categories: patients with NF2 and nontumor patients. The current criteria for an ABI in the United States are patients with NF2 12 years or older with poor hearing bilaterally and large vestibular schwannomas that do not allow for preservation of the cochlear nerve. In these patients, an ABI may be considered during first- or second-side tumor removal. The major benefit to implanting the ABI at the time of first tumor removal is to give the patient more time and experience using the device before they become reliant on it once their contralateral hearing decreases. Additionally, placement of the device may be more straightforward because of less anatomic distortion and scarring, which may occur over time and result in obscuring of brainstem landmarks.[20,21]

The nontumor indications for ABI include those with deafness secondary to bilateral temporal bone fractures in which the cochlear nerve has been avulsed or resulted in labyrinthine ossification, and in patients who suffered from meningitis that caused complete ossification of the cochlea. In addition, some patients with severe congenital inner ear malformation (eg, bilateral cochlear nerve deficiency/aplasia, cochlear aplasia, or complete labyrinthine aplasia) are only candidates for ABI because there is no receiving cavity to house a CI electrode array and/or a nerve to propagate the signal to the brainstem. Most experience with ABI in this cohort of patients stems from the international literature, and audiometric outcomes seem to be superior compared with those with NF2.[3,22]

Once a patient has met criteria for undergoing ABI surgery, thorough counseling with regards to expectations after implantation is critical. Patients should understand that an ABI does not provide normal sound quality and achieving open-set speech recognition is not achieved in most patients. Sound awareness may be a reasonable goal, however. Nevertheless, among the surgical risks, there are risks that the ABI fails to provide auditory sensations. Candidates should also understand the necessity of following through with postimplant speech/auditory rehabilitation to gain the maximum benefit from their implant.

Side selection is a highly individualized approach based on the patient's anatomy and cause of deafness. In general, the side with a more developed lateral recess is preferred. Also the side with more developed neuronal structures should be targeted because this may have implications for the degree of development of other structures inherent to the central auditory pathway. A high-riding jugular bulb may obstruct the view of the lateral recess because the cochlear nerve lies at a level that is inferior to the internal auditory canal, and should be evaluated on preoperative imaging. Lastly, in patients that have failed a trial of CI and are undergoing ABI, there is preliminary evidence that supports choosing the contralateral side because synergistic effects have been documented when both devices are used during the habilitation period.[23]

OPERATIVE TECHNIQUE

General anesthesia without long-term paralytics should be administered to allow for nerve monitoring. The patient is positioned in the supine position with the head turned to the contralateral side. Continuous electromyographic facial nerve monitor electrodes are applied in standard fashion. Subdermal electrodes are also placed for measuring an electrical auditory brainstem response (EABR) once the implant is in place. These electrodes are placed at the vertex of the head, over the seventh cervical vertebrae and the hairline of the occiput. An endotracheal tube with recurrent laryngeal nerve monitoring electrodes is also used for intubation to monitor cranial nerve X.

An ABI is placed using either a translabyrinthine approach or a retrosigmoid approach. In the NF2 population in which tumor removal is being performed simultaneously, a translabyrinthine approach is often preferred because it allows a more lateral view of the brainstem and a better view into the foramen of Luschka. If a retrosigmoid approach is performed, the craniotomy, skeletonizing, and retracting the sigmoid sinus anteriorly helps with providing direct access to the brainstem with the least cerebellar retraction.

After the skin is incised, an anteriorly based periosteal (Palva) flap is made and a superior/posterior subperiosteal pocket under the temporalis muscle is dissected. A bony well is drilled to secure the receiver/stimulator (**Fig. 2**A). A silicone replica of the receiver/stimulator is helpful in contouring the shape and size of the well. A trough between the receiver/stimulator and craniotomy opening is also drilled to house and protect the wires.

The approach to the cerebellopontine angle is performed in the standard fashion and the lower cranial nerves and CN VII and VIII (if present) are identified (**Fig. 2**B). If a remnant of CN VIII is present, this can be followed back to the brainstem. Otherwise, following CN IX from lateral to medial leads into the foramen of Luschka, which is the pathway to the cochlear nucleus intraoperatively. The foramen of Luschka projects into the cerebellopontine angle at the lateral border of the pontomedullary sulcus and is found between the roots of CN VII and CN IX. Dissection toward the brainstem involves displacing the flocculus followed by the choroid plexus dorsally and dividing the tenia choroidea (a soft tissue arachnoid band over the choroid plexus) to allow access to the foramen of Luschka (**Fig. 2**C, D). The dorsal surface of the brainstem is seen at this time. To verify correct identification of the lateral recess of the fourth ventricle a Valsalva is performed and CSF outflow should be noted.

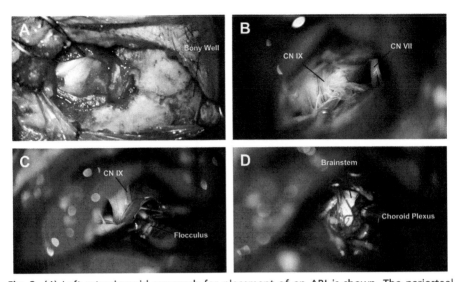

Fig. 2. (A) Left retrosigmoid approach for placement of an ABI is shown. The periosteal (Palva) flap is retracted anteriorly under fishhooks. The dura is anchored to the bone anteriorly retracting the sigmoid sinus. A bone flap has been removed and preserved on the back table for replacing at the end of the case. A bony well contoured to the shape of the device is drilled posteriorly and a trough that communicates with the craniotomy is created for placement of the electrode wires. A Telfa gauze is seen in the craniotomy defect, which was placed to prevent bone dust from entering intracranially while drilling the trough. (B) The initial approach to the brainstem is shown. In this patient, no vestibulocochlear nerve was identified confirming the diagnosis of cochlear nerve aplasia. The facial nerve was found in its usual location exiting the pontomedullary sulcus and running into an abnormal stenotic internal auditory canal. The nervus intermedius can also be seen. The lower cranial nerves are also identified encased in arachnoid. (C) The cerebellar flocculus is retracted dorsally and dissection proceeds from lateral to medial adjacent to CN IX. (D) The choroid plexus is identified and retracted dorsally and slightly superiorly to expose the foramen of Luschka and the brainstem.

The device is then brought onto the field and secured in the bony well and the soft tissue pocket is sutured closed to help prevent device migration (**Fig. 3**A). The lead wires are placed into a bony trough and the free ground wire is placed medial to the temporalis muscle periosteum. The Dacron wings on the electrode paddle may need to be carefully trimmed to allow proper positioning if the foramen is small. The paddle is inserted into the lateral recess of the fourth ventricle, just superior to where CN IX enters (**Fig. 3**B, C). The electrodes are oriented facing the brainstem and the paddle makes contact with the brainstem at the dorsal cochlear nucleus. The lack of surface landmarks makes identification of the exact location of cochlear nucleus difficult, and studies have shown high patient-to-patient variability in the position of the ABI electrode array.[24]

To aid with determining correct placement, audiologists are present intraoperatively to perform an EABR, which delivers single, biphasic pulses to the ABI array. The waveform generated can confirm stimulation of the cochlear nucleus and the morphology (eg, number of total peaks) may be predictive of postoperative auditory percepts.[25] The EABR is also important for determining whether nonauditory stimuli patterns are produced, such as facial nerve stimulation, myogenic responses, or changes in

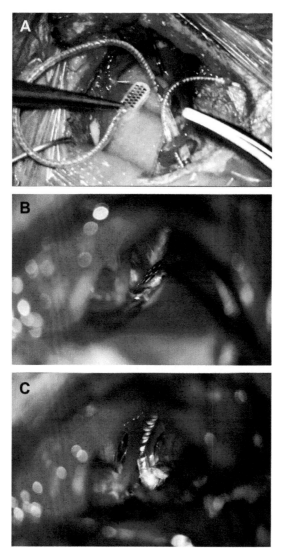

Fig. 3. (*A*) The device is then placed into the bony well and sutured tightly into place. Dacron wings along the paddle are trimmed. The lead wires are protected in a bony trough. The free ground wire is placed medial to the temporalis muscle. (*B*) The tip of the electrode paddle is being advanced into the foramen of Luschka. (*C*) The paddle is now fully advanced within the lateral recess of the fourth ventricle such that only the wire is visible and the electrodes are making contact with the brainstem at the dorsal cochlear nucleus. The relationship with CN IX is seen, which lies ventral to the foramen of Luschka.

pulse rate or hemodynamics, all of which may necessitate repositioning of the device or reprogramming.

Once the electrode is in appropriate position as confirmed by electrical testing, a piece of fat or Teflon felt is placed posterior to the electrode paddle to stabilize the device along the brainstem. The matrix of Dacron mesh on the electrode paddle provides a scaffold for ingrowth of fibrous tissue that further stabilizes the electrode position. The craniotomy is closed in standard fashion for the given approach.

Postoperatively, patients are monitored in the intensive care unit for 24 hours and subsequently transferred to the floor and begin mobilizing on postoperative day 1. Most patients are discharged home on postoperative day 3. The implant is activated 6 weeks after implantation. Special consideration is given for children during initial activation. Children are brought to the operating room and initial activation is done under general anesthesia with cranial nerve monitoring. Monitoring for vagal nerve stimulation and significant nonauditory side effects is performed because bradycardia, motor long tract stimulation, vertigo, throat tightening, and fainting may occur. For these reasons, cardiac monitoring and physician attendance are part of the protocol for initial stimulation in infants and children who are unable to communicate such feelings. The programming audiologist can "program out" any nonauditory symptoms that may occur.

The most common postoperative complications are CSF leak, implant migration, and nonauditory stimuli. CSF leaks may be treated with lumbar drain placement for CSF diversion. Rarely, reoperation for leak repair is necessary. Less common complications include cerebellar contusion, permanent facial palsy, meningitis, damage of the lower cranial nerves, hydrocephalus, pseudomeningocele, headache, and tinnitus. These complications are significantly less in the nontumor patients than in the NF2 population.[26]

OUTCOMES IN PATIENTS WITH NEUROFIBROMATOSIS TYPE 2

Auditory performance with ABIs remains highly variable. Although the speech outcomes are poorer compared with cochlear implantation, the restoration of some auditory input is encouraging. Variability in performance is attributable to variations in surgical technique, surgeon experience, postimplant programming, and signal-coding strategies. In addition, the tonotopic organization of the cochlear nucleus is much more complex than what is observed in the cochlea. Specifically, in the cochlear nucleus, frequencies are encoded from superficial-to-deep as opposed to along the surface, which is suboptimal for surface electrode stimulation.

Perhaps the most significant predictor of postoperative speech performance is related to the cause of the hearing loss, specifically whether it was caused by an NF2-related tumor versus a nontumor condition (eg, ossified cochlea, cochlear nerve avulsion from trauma). In patients with NF2, a multi-institutional study in the United States reported that overall (adults and children) 81% of implants received auditory sensations.[27] Unfortunately, this implies that nearly 20% fail to respond to stimulation altogether.[28,29] In addition, significant open-set word recognition is rare (around 10%) and therefore speech outcomes are much poorer with ABI compared with CI.[20,29,30] The greatest benefit attributable to the ABI comes in the form of enhanced lip reading, because it helps with determining the rhythm, stress, timing, and intensity of speech. When combined with lip reading, 93% of patients demonstrate improved sentence understanding at 3 to 6 months postimplant.[27]

OUTCOMES IN NONTUMOR PATIENTS

Outcomes in nontumor patients seem to be superior when compared with those with NF2.[22,31] Whereas only a small minority of patients with NF2 are capable of open-set sentence recognition, a significantly larger number of nontumor patients are able to achieve open-set speech perception. Colletti and colleagues[31] reported that postlingual adults without NF2 achieved an average of 59% open-set sentence recognition in the audition-alone mode, compared with 10% in patients with NF2.

These differences in auditory performance between patients with NF2 and those without tumors suggest that the NF2 condition itself may adversely affect the cochlear nucleus or auditory pathway. Although a large tumor may damage or distort the cochlear nucleus resulting in a poor outcome, this alone does not explain the discrepancy because even patients with small tumors that do not contact the brainstem have demonstrated poor performance.[32] Colletti and Shannon compared 10 patients with NF2 with 10 patients without NF2 and examined the electric stimulation thresholds, electrode selectivity, and amplitude modulation and speech perception.[22,31] They found that patients with NF2 had significantly worse modulation detection and speech discrimination than the non-NF2 cohorts. The physiologic reason for this is unclear but postulated to be caused by damage to a specific cell type or region within the cochlear nucleus.

OUTCOMES IN CHILDREN

It is estimated that 2.1% of all deaf children in the United State have bilateral cochlear or cochlear nerve aplasias, thereby making them ABI candidates.[33] Given the promising outcomes in non-NF2 ABI recipients, clinical trials involving ABI in children and infants who are not cochlear implant candidates are underway. A systematic review of 162 nontumor pediatric ABI patients found that the most common indication was cochlear nerve aplasia, accounting for 64% of patients. In this study, audiometric outcomes were noted to improve over time, such that at 5 years, almost 50% of patients were able to understand common phrases without lip reading.[34] Colletti and colleagues[7] reported on a long-term prospective analysis of 64 deaf children implanted with ABIs and followed for up to 12 years. All children in the study showed improvement in auditory perception, with 11% being able to converse on the telephone and 31.3% realizing open set speech recognition. A recent study by Asfour and colleagues[35] of 12 children with cochlear nerve deficiency who underwent ABI found that 11 patients achieved sound awareness. Of these 11 patients, four achieved greater than 50% accuracy on open set word discrimination and two achieved greater than 50% accuracy on closed set word discrimination. More encouraging were the positive scores on patient/parent-reported health-related quality-of-life surveys. Other experiences with pediatric ABI in the United States have also shown promise but long-term studies have not been published.[36,37]

SUMMARY

ABIs provide a safe and effective way to provide some degree of auditory rehabilitation to patients who are not candidates for a cochlear implant or who have failed to benefit from a cochlear implant. However, the degree of auditory rehabilitation can vary significantly and patients should be counseled with regards to realistic expectations and risks of the surgery. The functional aspect of hearing restored by ABIs is rarely comparable with the benefit received by most cochlear implant recipients. However, at present, ABIs are the only solution to providing auditory benefit to a group of patients who otherwise would be completely isolated from the auditory world. Ongoing research, including the use of light to stimulate genetically modified cells, known as optogenetics, and the fabrication of conformable electrode arrays that conform better to the complex surface of the brainstem are being investigated.[38] Future iterations of the ABI device design and signal processing strategies aim to further improve performance.

REFERENCES

1. Hitselberger WE, House WF, Edgerton BJ, et al. Cochlear nucleus implants. Otolaryngol Head Neck Surg 1984;92(1):52–4.
2. House WF, Hitselberger WE. Twenty-year report of the first auditory brain stem nucleus implant. Ann Otol Rhinol Laryngol 2001;110(2):103–4.
3. Colletti V, Carner M, Miorelli V, et al. Auditory brainstem implant (ABI): new frontiers in adults and children. Otolaryngol Head Neck Surg 2005;133(1): 126–38.
4. Grayeli AB, Bouccara D, Kalamarides M, et al. Auditory brainstem implant in bilateral and completely ossified cochleae. Otol Neurotol 2003;24(1): 79–82.
5. Colletti V, Carner M, Miorelli V, et al. Cochlear implantation at under 12 months: report on 10 patients. Laryngoscope 2005;115(3):445–9.
6. Colletti L. Beneficial auditory and cognitive effects of auditory brainstem implantation in children. Acta Otolaryngol 2007;127(9):943–6.
7. Colletti L, Shannon RV, Colletti V. The development of auditory perception in children after auditory brainstem implantation. Audiol Neurootol 2014;19(6): 386–94.
8. House Research Institute. FDA approves clinical trial of auditory brainstem implant procedure for children in U.S. Science Daily 2013. Available at: www. sciencedaily.com/releases/2013/01/130122101334.htm.
9. Lundin K, Stillesjo F, Nyberg G, et al. Self-reported benefit, sound perception, and quality-of-life in patients with auditory brainstem implants (ABIs). Acta Otolaryngol 2016;136(1):62–7.
10. Fernandes NF, Goffi-Gomez MV, Magalhaes AT, et al. Satisfaction and quality of life in users of auditory brainstem implant. Codas 2017;29(2):e20160059.
11. Otto SR, Shannon RV, Wilkinson EP, et al. Audiologic outcomes with the penetrating electrode auditory brainstem implant. Otol Neurotol 2008;29(8): 1147–54.
12. Buchman CA, Teagle HF, Roush PA, et al. Cochlear implantation in children with labyrinthine anomalies and cochlear nerve deficiency: implications for auditory brainstem implantation. Laryngoscope 2011;121(9):1979–88.
13. Warren FM 3rd, Wiggins RH 3rd, Pitt C, et al. Apparent cochlear nerve aplasia: to implant or not to implant? Otol Neurotol 2010;31(7):1088–94.
14. Song MH, Kim SC, Kim J, et al. The cochleovestibular nerve identified during auditory brainstem implantation in patients with narrow internal auditory canals: can preoperative evaluation predict cochleovestibular nerve deficiency? Laryngoscope 2011;121(8):1773–9.
15. Roehm PC, Mallen-St Clair J, Jethanamest D, et al. Auditory rehabilitation of patients with neurofibromatosis type 2 by using cochlear implants. J Neurosurg 2011;115(4):827–34.
16. Peng KA, Lorenz MB, Otto SR, et al. Cochlear implantation and auditory brainstem implantation in neurofibromatosis type 2. Laryngoscope 2018;128(9): 2163–9.
17. Neff BA, Wiet RM, Lasak JM, et al. Cochlear implantation in the neurofibromatosis type 2 patient: long-term follow-up. Laryngoscope 2007;117(6):1069–72.
18. Pai I, Dhar V, Kelleher C, et al. Cochlear implantation in patients with vestibular schwannoma: a single United Kingdom center experience. Laryngoscope 2013;123(8):2019–23.

19. Carlson ML, Breen JT, Driscoll CL, et al. Cochlear implantation in patients with neurofibromatosis type 2: variables affecting auditory performance. Otol Neurotol 2012;33(5):853–62.
20. Brackmann DE, Hitselberger WE, Nelson RA, et al. Auditory brainstem implant: I. Issues in surgical implantation. Otolaryngol Head Neck Surg 1993;108(6): 624–33.
21. Colletti V, Sacchetto L, Giarbini N, et al. Retrosigmoid approach for auditory brainstem implant. J Laryngol Otol Suppl 2000;(27):37–40.
22. Colletti V, Shannon RV. Open set speech perception with auditory brainstem implant? Laryngoscope 2005;115(11):1974–8.
23. Friedmann DR, Asfour L, Shapiro WH, et al. Performance with an auditory brainstem implant and contralateral cochlear implant in pediatric patients. Audiol Neurootol 2018;23(4):216–21.
24. Barber SR, Kozin ED, Remenschneider AK, et al. Auditory brainstem implant array position varies widely among adult and pediatric patients and is associated with perception. Ear Hear 2017;38(6):e343–51.
25. Anwar A, Singleton A, Fang Y, et al. The value of intraoperative EABRs in auditory brainstem implantation. Int J Pediatr Otorhinolaryngol 2017;101:158–63.
26. Colletti V, Shannon RV, Carner M, et al. Complications in auditory brainstem implant surgery in adults and children. Otol Neurotol 2010;31(4):558–64.
27. Ebinger K, Otto S, Arcaroli J, et al. Multichannel auditory brainstem implant: US clinical trial results. J Laryngol Otol Suppl 2000;(27):50–3.
28. Schwartz MS, Otto SR, Shannon RV, et al. Auditory brainstem implants. Neurotherapeutics 2008;5(1):128–36.
29. Otto SR, Brackmann DE, Hitselberger WE, et al. Multichannel auditory brainstem implant: update on performance in 61 patients. J Neurosurg 2002;96(6): 1063–71.
30. Toh EH, Luxford WM. Cochlear and brainstem implantation. Otolaryngol Clin North Am 2002;35(2):325–42.
31. Colletti V, Shannon R, Carner M, et al. Outcomes in nontumor adults fitted with the auditory brainstem implant: 10 years' experience. Otol Neurotol 2009;30(5): 614–8.
32. Behr R, Colletti V, Matthies C, et al. New outcomes with auditory brainstem implants in NF2 patients. Otol Neurotol 2014;35(10):1844–51.
33. Kaplan AB, Kozin ED, Puram SV, et al. Auditory brainstem implant candidacy in the United States in children 0-17 years old. Int J Pediatr Otorhinolaryngol 2015; 79(3):310–5.
34. Noij KS, Kozin ED, Sethi R, et al. Systematic review of nontumor pediatric auditory brainstem implant outcomes. Otolaryngol Head Neck Surg 2015;153(5): 739–50.
35. Asfour L, Friedmann DR, Shapiro WH, et al. Early experience and health related quality of life outcomes following auditory brainstem implantation in children. Int J Pediatr Otorhinolaryngol 2018;113:140–9.
36. Puram SV, Barber SR, Kozin ED, et al. Outcomes following pediatric auditory brainstem implant surgery: early experiences in a North American center. Otolaryngol Head Neck Surg 2016;155(1):133–8.
37. Wilkinson EP, Eisenberg LS, Krieger MD, et al. Initial results of a safety and feasibility study of auditory brainstem implantation in congenitally deaf children. Otol Neurotol 2017;38(2):212–20.
38. Wong K, Kozin ED, Kanumuri VV, et al. Auditory brainstem implants: recent progress and future perspectives. Front Neurosci 2019;13:10.

Vestibular Implantation and the Feasibility of Fluoroscopy-Guided Electrode Insertion

Joost Johannes Antonius Stultiens, MD[a],
Alida Annechien Postma, MD, PhD[b], Nils Guinand, MD, PhD[c],
Angélica Pérez Fornos, PhD[c], Hermanus Kingma, PhD[a],
Raymond van de Berg, MD, PhD[a],*

KEYWORDS

- Bilateral vestibulopathy • Vestibular implant • Implanted Electrodes • Implanted
- Semicircular canals • Radiography • Fluoroscopy • Feasibility study
- Proof of concept study

KEY POINTS

- The vestibular implant aims to restore loss of vestibular function.
- First results in humans show that the vestibular implant is feasible as a therapeutic device in the near future.
- The intralabyrinthine surgical approach is currently being investigated by multiple groups, but it entails the challenge of correct electrode placement.
- Fluoroscopy may improve electrode placement during vestibular implantation.

INTRODUCTION

Bilateral vestibulopathy, a severe bilateral function loss of the vestibular organs, nerves, or a combination of both, is often disabling.[1,2] It is a heterogeneous disorder with different etiologies, varying from ototoxicity (eg, gentamicin) to meningitis,

Disclosures: None.
[a] Department of Otorhinolaryngology–Head and Neck Surgery, School for Mental Health and Neuroscience, Faculty of Health Medicine and Life Sciences, P.O. box 5800, 6202 AZ, Maastricht University Medical Center, Maastricht, The Netherlands; [b] Department of Radiology and Nuclear Medicine, School for Mental Health and Neuroscience, Faculty of Health Medicine and Life Sciences, P.O. box 5800, 6202 AZ, Maastricht University Medical Center, Maastricht, The Netherlands; [c] Division of Otorhinolaryngology-Head and Neck Surgery, Department of Clinical Neurosciences, Geneva University Hospitals, Rue Gabrielle-Perret-Gentil 4, 1205, Geneva, Switzerland
* Corresponding author.
E-mail address: raymond.vande.berg@mumc.nl

Otolaryngol Clin N Am 53 (2020) 115–126
https://doi.org/10.1016/j.otc.2019.09.006
oto.theclinics.com
0030-6665/20/© 2019 The Author(s). Published by Elsevier Inc. This is an open access article under the CC BY license (http://creativecommons.org/licenses/by/4.0/).

genetic, autoimmune, neurodegenerative (eg, ataxia), and other diseases. However, in up to half of the cases, the cause remains idiopathic.[3] Bilateral vestibulopathy can lead to many symptoms, including imbalance and oscillopsia (the illusory movement of the environment).[4,5] It has a socioeconomic impact,[6] reduces quality of life,[7] and increases risk of falling up to 31 times.[6] It is estimated that more than 3 million people are affected, but this is likely to be underestimated because of many diagnostic challenges.[8] Unfortunately, current treatment options, such as physiotherapy, often have a low yield and bilateral vestibulopathy cannot yet be sufficiently treated in most of the cases.[9]

Therefore, research groups around the world have investigated the feasibility of an artificial balance organ: the vestibular implant (VI). The VI is in concept analogous to the cochlear implant. Instead of sound, it captures motion using gyroscopes. This motion information is then transferred to a processor that converts it into electrical signals. Subsequently, electrodes implanted in the vicinity of the ampullar branches of the vestibular nerve are used to convey these electrical signals and stimulate the vestibular nerves. By this, motion information is transferred to the brain.[10] Until now, only stimulation of the semicircular canals has been reported in humans (**Box 1**), although otolith stimulation is also being investigated. The Geneva-Maastricht group was the first group to implant humans with a fully functional VI. This group was able to show the feasibility of a VI in humans[10] and various findings were reported. First, it was possible to elicit an electrically evoked vestibulo-ocular reflex in the plane of the stimulated canal, and (partially) restore vestibular function in the low and high frequencies of movement.[11,12] However, the vestibulo-ocular reflex was not always aligned with the stimulated canal, because of current spread to the other canals and/or otolith organs.[10] Second, the brain was able to adapt to the baseline stimulation, while still reacting on motion-induced modulation of the implant.[10] Third, the characteristics of the electrically evoked vestibulo-ocular reflex mimicked those of the natural vestibulo-ocular reflex.[13] Fourth, it was possible to also elicit vestibulocollic and vestibulospinal reflexes, recorded by vestibular evoked myogenic potentials and

---

Box 1
Overview VI research in humans

Potential indications (current and future)
- Bilateral vestibular loss
- Incomplete centrally compensated unilateral labyrinthine hypofunction
- Fluctuating vestibular hypofunction (ie, "pacemaker" to treat vertigo attacks)

Design
    Gyroscopes, external processor, and implanted stimulator connected to electrode leads close to the vestibular nerve

Surgical approaches
- Intralabyrinthine: one electrode lead in each semicircular canal
- Extralabyrinthine: electrode leads directly on the nerves, outside semicircular canals

Main findings of the VI in humans
- The vestibulo-ocular reflex can (partially) be restored
- The brain adapts to baseline stimulation, while still responding to motion-modulated stimulation
- The electrically evoked vestibulo-ocular reflex (partially) mimics the natural reflex
- The vestibulocollic reflex is elicited, and controlled postural responses are generated
- Vestibular sensations are elicited, but these perceptions are highly variable
- The vestibular implant can overrule natural vestibular function
- Dynamic visual abilities are restored during walking and during fast head movements

change of posture, respectively.[14] Fifth, perception of input from the VI varied: not always vertigo or rotatory sensations were reported, but also other percepts, such as sounds or pressure.[10] Sixth, VI information was able to overrule the residual natural vestibular information, where the brain behaved nonlinearly. This might pave the way for using the VI as a "vestibular pacemaker" in case of fluctuating vestibular function, such as vertigo attacks.[15,16] Finally, a functional benefit was demonstrated by reducing oscillopsia and improving vision during walking on a treadmill[17] and during fast head movements.[18]

Given these results, it can be hypothesized that indications for the VI might not only remain restricted to bilateral vestibulopathy in the future. Other indications include: uncompensated unilateral vestibular hypofunction, presbyvestibulopathy,[19] and therapy resistant vertigo attacks.[15,16,20] However, still many challenges are met in VI research. One major challenge is refining vestibular implantation surgery, to lower risks of hearing loss and to get optimal electrode placement. Two types of surgery were developed: the extralabyrinthine approach and the intralabyrinthine approach.[21–23] With the extralabyrinthine approach, the electrodes are placed outside the labyrinth. Under local anesthesia, the nerves are directly approached and electrodes are placed onto the ampullar branches of the vestibular nerves. Because the labyrinth is not opened, the risk of sensorineural hearing loss is minimized. However, it is a challenging surgery (eg, higher risk of damaging the facial nerve) that requires extensive training. Furthermore, electrode fixation is difficult.[10,21–23] Therefore, the intralabyrinthine approach is nowadays preferred by most groups.[10,24,25] With the intralabyrinthine approach, the semicircular canals are fenestrated close to the ampulla, because previous research showed optimal stimulation near the ampullary nerves.[26] Therefore, electrodes are inserted as close as possible to these nerves. However, by opening the inner ear, the risk of sensorineural hearing loss increases. Previously, implantation of the vestibular system by another group resulted in postoperative sensorineural loss in their population.[24] Because many patients with bilateral vestibulopathy still have sufficient hearing,[3] it is important that research focuses on hearing preservation during vestibular implantation surgery. Fortunately, it was shown that electrode insertion of the semicircular canals is possible without acutely changing the auditory function as measured with auditory brainstem response.[27] Nevertheless because of ethical reasons, the Geneva-Maastricht group currently only implants patients with bilateral vestibulopathy who are already deaf in the ear to be implanted.[10]

Next to hearing preservation, it is challenging to get the electrode as close as possible to the ampullary nerve (in the ampullae of the semicircular canals) using the intralabyrinthine approach. After all, when the semicircular canal is fenestrated, the sensory epithelium is often not directly visible. It is not preferred to widely open the fenestration until the sensory epithelium is reached, because this might induce hearing loss.[28] This implies that the electrode is inserted "blindly," without the surgeon knowing exactly how far the electrode needs to be inserted, to make close contact with the sensory epithelium of the ampullary nerve. As a result, electrode position was previously not always optimal.[29] Therefore, there is a need to optimize electrode placement during surgery. Several options have been explored to facilitate proper electrode positioning, but none of them have proven to be infallible: (1) vestibular evoked compound action potentials might be of benefit, but similarly to cochlear implantation, they are not always obtained during vestibular implantation surgery[30]; (2) surgical landmarks show too many interindividual differences to get a precise position in a large group of individuals[31]; (3) vestibulo-ocular reflex testing to verify the position of the electrodes is compromised by general anesthesia[32]; and (4) additional electrodes on the electrode lead might increase the chance of hitting the target,[24,25,31] but do not guarantee proper positioning. One of the possibilities to improve electrode positioning is real-time visual guidance of electrode insertion. Multiple imaging techniques can potentially aid electrode insertion but each have their own pros and cons.[33] Preliminary studies by the Geneva-Maastricht group demonstrated that high-frequency ultrasound and optical coherence tomography have a superior image quality, but often lack the ability to penetrate the bony labyrinth deep enough to visualize the ampullae of the semicircular canals. Therefore, imaging techniques containing better penetration properties were considered.

Fluoroscopy is an imaging technique that captures moving images in real-time using x-rays. The x-ray technique was developed in 1895[34] and within a few months fluoroscopes became commercially available. Soon after its availability, it already proved useful in otolaryngologic practice.[35,36] Although nowadays many advanced imaging techniques are used in otolaryngology, fluoroscopy is still an important technique in daily practice of many medical specialties requiring real-time guidance. Its utility in cochlear implantation is still being investigated, but studies suggest that it may be useful in challenging cases, such as abnormal cochlear anatomy.[37–39] This technique can clearly display the structures of the inner ear and cochlear implant electrodes during surgery.[37,38] Considering the similarities with VI surgery, fluoroscopy could possibly overcome the blind insertion in this procedure.

With this background provided on the VI, the aim of this work is to demonstrate the potential of fluoroscopy-guidance in the intralabyrinthine surgical approach, to correctly place the three VI electrodes in the semicircular canals. It was hypothesized that the semicircular canal ampullae and electrode leads could be identified and that the insertion could be improved using real-time visual guidance by fluoroscopy.

MATERIALS AND METHODS: INVESTIGATIONS OF FLUOROSCOPY-ASSISTED VESTIBULAR IMPLANTATION
Subjects and Preparation

Formalin-fixed cadaveric human heads with intact skull from donor subjects were included. A canal-wall up mastoidectomy was performed bilaterally and the semicircular canals were skeletonized. Subsequently, a single fenestration of approximately 0.7 to 1 mm was made in each bony semicircular canal: the lateral semicircular canal was fenestrated near the tip of the short process of the incus, the posterior semicircular canal was fenestrated at the intersection with Donaldson line, and the superior semicircular canal was fenestrated at an estimated similar distance from its ampulla as the lateral semicircular canal fenestration.

Surgical Set-Up

The cadaveric head was placed on a computed tomography (CT) scan table, rotated away from the surgeon (30°). A Ziehm Vision RFD three-dimensional (3D) mobile fluoroscopy unit (Ziehm Imaging GmbH, Nürnberg, Germany) was used to visualize the semicircular canal ampullae. This C-arm encompasses a 3D functionality, but for this experiment only the two-dimensional functionality was used. Based on preliminary findings to optimize semicircular canal visualization, the C-arm was arranged in a modified Stenvers position: from orbitomeatal plane 10° craniocaudal and 30° left anterior oblique (right ear) or 30° right anterior oblique (left ear). If necessary, the C-arm was slightly adjusted until all ampullae (superior, lateral, posterior) were visualized in the same image.

Implanting the Semicircular Canals

The aim was to position the electrode tips as close as possible to the center of the semicircular canal ampullae. First, the electrodes were blindly inserted using silicone electrodes (ø0.6 mm) with an enclosed platinium-irididium wire of ø0.5 μm (MED-EL, Innsbruck, Austria), until the estimated position of each electrode tip was in the ampulla of the inserted canal. This way, radiation exposure could be minimized to only the visualization and repositioning procedure. Then, fluoroscopy was used to visualize the electrode and adjust its position. The optimum location of the electrode tip (ie, the center of the ampulla of the inserted semicircular canal) in the fluoroscopy images was determined by a radiologist (AP) and an ear, nose, throat surgeon (RvdB) in consensus. Both persons cooperated together with the surgeon performing the implantations (JS) in placing the electrode tips in their final positions. Directly after implanting the three semicircular canals, a CT scan of the head was performed with a slice thickness of 0.4 mm using Somatom Force CT (Siemens, Forchheim, Germany) to determine the final position of the insertion. The whole procedure was repeated for the contralateral ear.

Analysis

The CT scan images were used for image analysis. Because each head was implanted on both sides subsequently, each head was scanned twice (after implanting each side) and thus two scans were available of each inner ear: one with and one without electrodes implanted. The two CT scans of each head were manually aligned using the open source software 3D Slicer version 4.8.[40] Then, automated fusing using the BRAINSFit registration algorithm[41] was applied, as previously described.[42] The unimplanted ear of each scan was manually segmented and a 3D model was created (**Fig. 1**A). Based on the CT images and the 3D model, a fiducial was placed at the center of the ampulla of each semicircular canal (**Fig. 1**B). This was explicitly not performed in the scan with electrodes, to avoid confounding caused by the electrode tip position (eg, placing the fiducial closer to the electrode tip). Separately, in the implanted ear of each scan, fiducials were placed at the electrode tips (**Fig. 1**C).

Because of the previous alignment of the CT scans, the distances between the fiducials in the centers of the ampullae and the corresponding electrode tips could be calculated in 3D Euclidean space (**Fig. 1**D). Median distances were determined. Additionally, a distance less than 1.5 mm was defined as correct electrode placement. This was based on the fact that stimulation of the ampullae seems to be most effective,[26] and that the average diameter of an ampulla is approximately 1.5 to 2 mm (height-length).[43]

Additionally, these obtained distances were compared with previously reported mean distances from blindly inserted electrodes in humans.[29] The Mann-Whitney U test was used to test for differences between the two insertion techniques (all placements of fluoroscopy-guided vs blind insertion). The proportions of correctly placed electrodes (ie, <1.5 mm) were calculated for both techniques, and the 95% confidence intervals (CI) were calculated using Wilson score interval.

Ethics

This study was performed by virtue of three donors. Handwritten and signed codicils from the donors are kept at the Department of Anatomy and Embryology, according to the Dutch Corpse Disposal Act ("Wet op de lijkbezorging", 1991). The procedures in this investigation were in accordance with legislation and ethical standards in the Netherlands.

RESULTS

Six ears from three donors were sequentially implanted, guided by fluoroscopy, and underwent CT scanning. Fluoroscopic visualization of the ampulla and real-time visual

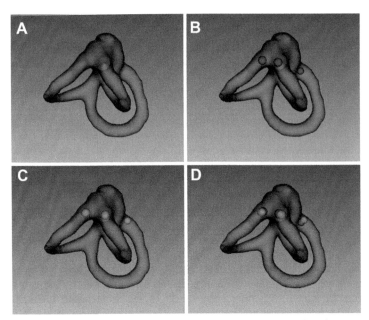

Fig. 1. Process of image analysis. (*A*) Result of image segmentation. (*B*) Placement of fiducials at the center of the semicircular canal ampullae, based on the CT scan before implantation. (*C*) Placement of fiducials at electrode tips, based on the postimplantation CT scan. (*D*) Integration of all fiducials based on the fusion of the two CT scans, on which the distances of the electrode tips to the center of the ampullae could be calculated.

guidance of electrode insertion was possible in all 18 semicircular canals. The ampulla was visible as a widening of the inner border of the bony semicircular canal, adjacent to the vestibule (**Fig. 2**). After the first blind insertion, all electrodes were adjusted using fluoroscopy. The distance between the center of the ampulla and the electrode tip is presented for all semicircular canals in **Table 1**. The biggest deviation from the target location was 2.0 mm. The median distances for the superior, lateral, and posterior semicircular canal were 0.60 mm, 0.85 mm, and 0.65 mm, respectively (**Fig. 3**). The proportions of correctly placed electrodes were 100% for superior and lateral semicircular canal and 83% for the posterior semicircular canal. All semicircular canals taken together, the median distance was 0.7 mm (interquartile range, 0.5–1.0 mm), and 94% of the electrodes (95% CI, 74%–99%) was placed correctly (bold in **Table 1**).

Comparison of the current data with the blind insertion technique (based on the raw data from Nguyen and colleagues[29]) showed that the electrode tips of the fluoroscopy-guided insertion technique were significantly closer to their target ($P = .01$). After all, the blind insertion technique resulted in 75% correctly placed electrodes (95% CI, 47%–91%), with an overall median distance of 1.2 mm (minimum 0.4 mm; maximum 5.3 mm).

DISCUSSION

This work reviewed a comprehensive list of indications for vestibular implantation and some of the basic concepts that underlie this new cranial nerve implant. Specifically, the feasibility and utility of fluoroscopy as an imaging technique to provide real-time visual guidance during intralabyrinthine vestibular implantation was investigated. All

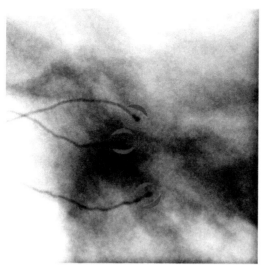

Fig. 2. Fluoroscopy image of a right ear with implanted electrodes (Ear #4) in the superior, lateral, and posterior semicircular canal (*top-bottom*). *Red lines* indicate the ampullae.

electrode tips were placed close to their intended target location. This was significantly closer than previously described with blind insertion.[29] Overall in this study, 94% of the electrodes were correctly inserted (ie, <1.5-mm distance), compared with 75% with blind insertion. Therefore, these results suggest that fluoroscopy may aid adequate electrode placement during vestibular implantation.

Although promising, still some challenges are met when applying fluoroscopy for vestibular implantation. One of the challenges in fluoroscopy-guided implantation is to sufficiently visualize the ampullae of the semicircular canals. With the applied position of the C-arm in the modified Stenvers plane described previously, the resulting image was deemed optimal for simultaneous visualization of all three semicircular canals. This configuration is almost perpendicular to the lateral and superior semicircular canals, but not perpendicular to the posterior canal. This made it more difficult to determine the ampullar region of the posterior semicircular canal, also because of

Table 1
Distances of electrode tips from intended target locations (center of ampullae)

| | Ear | Distance (mm) | | |
		Superior SCC	Lateral SCC	Posterior SCC
1	Left	0.9	0.6	0.8
2	Right	0.5	0.7	0.5
3	Left	0.3	1.2	2.0*
4	Right	0.2	1.0	0.5
5	Right	0.7	0.6	1.4
6	Left	0.9	1.1	0.0

* Except this, all other values indicates correctly placed electrodes in the SCCs according to the predetermined criteria (ie, <1.5-mm distance).
   Abbreviation: SCC, semicircular canal.

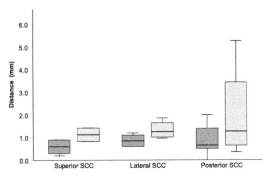

Fig. 3. Distribution of distances (mm) from the tip of the electrode to the center of the ampulla, per semicircular canal, for the fluoroscopy-guided insertion technique (*left-sided dark gray bars*; this study) and for the blind insertion technique (*right-sided light gray bars*; derived from Nguyen and colleagues). (*Data from* Nguyen TAK, Cavuscens S, Ranieri M, et al. Characterization of Cochlear, Vestibular and Cochlear-Vestibular Electrically Evoked Compound Action Potentials in Patients with a Vestibulo-Cochlear Implant. *Front Neurosci.* 2017;11:645.)

overprojection of other structures of the temporal bone. This probably also explains why electrode distances in this canal showed the widest variability, although half of the electrode tips were within 0.5 mm of the target. Other configurations of the C-arm were tried in a preliminary study, including a separate configuration for the visualization of the posterior semicircular canal, but they did not yield better visualization than the modified Stenvers plane. Second, taking this into account, applying fluoroscopy for vestibular implantation requires training to correctly position the C-arm and to interpret the fluoroscopy images. The total dose is influenced by the duration of exposure, the number of images per second, the required quality of the images, and the field size. If the team is able to swiftly set up the C-arm to obtain images in the modified Stenvers plane, this also reduces radiation dose because exposure during repositioning is limited and a narrowed beam can be applied. Because this involved a feasibility study, and limited training of the team was performed, administered radiation dose was not yet taken into account. However, studies investigating the use of fluoroscopy in cochlear implantation surgery estimated that with modern fluoroscopy devices, the total doses stay well lower than recommended total exposure limits.[37,38] Third, a previous study with a virtual model of the rhesus monkey labyrinth, showed that the electrodes closest to the crista produce the greatest nerve fiber activity recruitment with the lowest thresholds.[26] Therefore it was assumed that electrodes should be positioned as close as possible to the sensory epithelium of the ampullary nerves, which are not visible with fluoroscopy. These structures are actually not located in the centers of the ampullae, but in the ampullary walls.[44] However, because vestibular electrodes are not yet fully designed to hug the walls of the ampullae, it was not possible to reproducibly position the electrodes against these walls. Therefore for this study, it was chosen to use the centers of the ampullae as the target locations. After electrode design modifications, electrode contact with the sensory epithelium could be tested in the future. The inability to visualize this epithelium with fluoroscopy is not expected to be a drawback, because the ampullary walls (its primary location) are clearly visible with fluoroscopy. Lastly, it seemed that of the 18 inserted electrodes, one electrode was inserted greater than 1.5 mm too far off the center of the ampulla (Ear #3, PSCC, 2.0 mm). This electrode turned out to be inserted too deep into the canal, almost reaching into the vestibule. However, with multiple electrodes on the lead[31] and the right selection of the stimulating electrode postoperatively, stimulation could still take place in close proximity to the target.

The following approach is advised for further investigations: before fenestration of the semicircular canals, optimize the fluoroscopic visualization (ie, adequate window and angles in craniocaudal and left/right plane); after fenestration, insert the electrodes blindly; then, adjust the position of the electrodes using fluoroscopy. This approach confines the administered radiation dosage while also limiting electrode manipulation. Further research should investigate the value of this technique in the operation room in a larger patient group, before definite conclusions about its benefit in VI surgery can be drawn.

Limitations

The fiducials used for calculating the distances from electrode tip to ampulla were placed manually. This could have introduced a bias, especially for determining the centers of the ampullae. However, observer bias was minimized by determining this target position on the CT scan without inserted electrodes and fusing these images with the postimplantation images. Still, one drawback of the fusion is an inaccuracy of the alignment. Because the misalignment can occur in every direction, this may lead to an underestimation of correctly placed electrodes, although this inaccuracy is on average only 0.05 to 0.16 mm.[42] Furthermore, because of the small sample size, only descriptive statistics were applied. No predictions can be made regarding the robustness of the results (eg, the relationship with patient characteristics).

SUMMARY

Vestibular implantation is an emerging technology that offers direct cranial nerve stimulation for bilateral vestibulopathy and potentially other vestibular disorders. Although there are still challenges to overcome in the development of this device and its implantation technique, research demonstrates feasibility and utility of the VI to improve clinical outcomes for patients with certain vestibular disorders that do not respond to traditional therapies. This article showed that fluoroscopy can provide the VI- surgeon with direct feedback on the location of the VI electrodes and consequently improve correct electrode placement. A future trial should validate this approach in a larger patient group, before its clinical value can be determined.

FUNDING:

This work was supported by MED-EL (Innsbruck, Austria; grant number FK3250). The funders had no role in study design, data collection, data analysis, interpretation of data, decision to publish, or preparation of the manuscript.

ACKNOWLEDGMENTS

The authors thank the people who donated their body for dissection in the interest of science and education. Furthermore, they thank Audrey Moonen, Peter Fijten, and Maaike Bosma for assisting as radiologic technicians during the experiments and the Department of Anatomy and Embryology at Maastricht University for their assistance and care for the cadavers.

REFERENCES

1. Ward BK, Agrawal Y, Hoffman HJ, et al. Prevalence and impact of bilateral vestibular hypofunction: results from the 2008 US National Health Interview Survey. JAMA Otolaryngol Head Neck Surg 2013;139(8):803–10.
2. Hain TC, Cherchi M, Yacovino DA. Bilateral vestibular loss. Semin Neurol 2013; 33(3):195–203.
3. Lucieer F, Vonk P, Guinand N, et al. Bilateral vestibular hypofunction: insights in etiologies, clinical subtypes, and diagnostics. Front Neurol 2016;7:26.
4. Lucieer F, Duijn S, Van Rompaey V, et al. Full spectrum of reported symptoms of bilateral vestibulopathy needs further investigation-a systematic review. Front Neurol 2018;9:352.
5. Strupp M, Kim JS, Murofushi T, et al. Bilateral vestibulopathy: diagnostic criteria consensus document of the Classification Committee of the Barany Society. J Vestib Res 2017;27(4):177–89.
6. Sun DQ, Ward BK, Semenov YR, et al. Bilateral vestibular deficiency: quality of life and economic implications. JAMA Otolaryngol Head Neck Surg 2014; 140(6):527–34.
7. Guinand N, Boselie F, Guyot JP, et al. Quality of life of patients with bilateral vestibulopathy. Ann Otol Rhinol Laryngol 2012;121(7):471–7.
8. van de Berg R, van Tilburg M, Kingma H. Bilateral vestibular hypofunction: challenges in establishing the diagnosis in adults. ORL J Otorhinolaryngol Relat Spec 2015;77(4):197–218.
9. Porciuncula F, Johnson CC, Glickman LB. The effect of vestibular rehabilitation on adults with bilateral vestibular hypofunction: a systematic review. J Vestib Res 2012;22(5–6):283–98.
10. Guinand N, van de Berg R, Cavuscens S, et al. Vestibular implants: 8 years of experience with electrical stimulation of the vestibular nerve in 11 patients with bilateral vestibular loss. ORL J Otorhinolaryngol Relat Spec 2015;77(4):227–40.
11. Perez Fornos A, Guinand N, van de Berg R, et al. Artificial balance: restoration of the vestibulo-ocular reflex in humans with a prototype vestibular neuroprosthesis. Front Neurol 2014;5:66.
12. Guinand N, Van de Berg R, Cavuscens S, et al. The video head impulse test to assess the efficacy of vestibular implants in humans. Front Neurol 2017;8:600.
13. van de Berg R, Guinand N, Nguyen TA, et al. The vestibular implant: frequency-dependency of the electrically evoked vestibulo-ocular reflex in humans. Front Syst Neurosci 2014;8:255.
14. Fornos AP, van de Berg R, Armand S, et al. Cervical myogenic potentials and controlled postural responses elicited by a prototype vestibular implant. J Neurol 2019;266(Suppl 1):33–41.
15. van de Berg R, Guinand N, Ranieri M, et al. The vestibular implant input interacts with residual natural function. Front Neurol 2017;8:644.
16. Rubinstein JT, Bierer S, Kaneko C, et al. Implantation of the semicircular canals with preservation of hearing and rotational sensitivity: a vestibular neurostimulator suitable for clinical research. Otol Neurotol 2012;33(5):789–96.
17. Guinand N, Van de Berg R, Cavuscens S, et al. Restoring visual acuity in dynamic conditions with a vestibular implant. Front Neurosci 2016;10:577.
18. Starkov D, Guinand N, Lucieer F, et al. Restoring the high-frequency dynamic visual acuity with a vestibular implant prototype in humans. Audiol Neurootol. In press.

19. Agrawal Y, Van de Berg R, Wuyts F, et al. Presbyvestibulopathy: diagnostic criteria consensus document of the classification committee of the Barany Society. J Vestib Res 2019;29(4):161–70.
20. van de Berg R, Guinand N, Stokroos RJ, et al. The vestibular implant: quo vadis? Front Neurol 2011;2:47.
21. Wall C 3rd, Kos MI, Guyot JP. Eye movements in response to electric stimulation of the human posterior ampullary nerve. Ann Otol Rhinol Laryngol 2007;116(5):369–74.
22. Guyot JP, Sigrist A, Pelizzone M, et al. Eye movements in response to electrical stimulation of the lateral and superior ampullary nerves. Ann Otol Rhinol Laryngol 2011;120(2):81–7.
23. van de Berg R, Guinand N, Guyot JP, et al. The modified ampullar approach for vestibular implant surgery: feasibility and its first application in a human with a long-term vestibular loss. Front Neurol 2012;3:18.
24. Phillips JO, Ling L, Nie K, et al. Vestibular implantation and longitudinal electrical stimulation of the semicircular canal afferents in human subjects. J Neurophysiol 2015;113(10):3866–92.
25. Chiang B, Fridman GY, Dai C, et al. Design and performance of a multichannel vestibular prosthesis that restores semicircular canal sensation in rhesus monkey. IEEE Trans Neural Syst Rehabil Eng 2011;19(5):588–98.
26. Hedjoudje A, Hayden R, Dai C, et al. Virtual rhesus labyrinth model predicts responses to electrical stimulation delivered by a vestibular prosthesis. J Assoc Res Otolaryngol 2019;20(4):313–39.
27. van de Berg R, Lucieer F, Guinand N, et al. The vestibular implant: hearing preservation during intralabyrinthine electrode insertion-a case report. Front Neurol 2017;8:137.
28. Parnes LS, McClure JA. Posterior semicircular canal occlusion in the normal hearing ear. Otolaryngol Head Neck Surg 1991;104(1):52–7.
29. Nguyen TAK, Cavuscens S, Ranieri M, et al. Characterization of cochlear, vestibular and cochlear-vestibular electrically evoked compound action potentials in patients with a vestibulo-cochlear implant. Front Neurosci 2017;11:645.
30. Nie K, Bierer SM, Ling L, et al. Characterization of the electrically evoked compound action potential of the vestibular nerve. Otol Neurotol 2011;32(1):88–97.
31. Seppen BF, van Hoof M, Stultiens JJA, et al. Drafting a surgical procedure using a computational anatomy driven approach for precise, robust, and safe vestibular neuroprosthesis placement-when one size does not fit all. Otol Neurotol 2019;40(5S Suppl 1):S51–8.
32. Poon CC, Irwin MG. Anaesthesia for deep brain stimulation and in patients with implanted neurostimulator devices. Br J Anaesth 2009;103(2):152–65.
33. Bance M, Zarowski A, Adamson RA, et al. New imaging modalities in otology. Adv Otorhinolaryngol 2018;81:1–13.
34. Röntgen CW. Ueber eine neue Art von Strahlen. Würzburg (Germany): Stahel; 1895.
35. Macintyre J. Röntgen rays in laryngeal surgery. The Journal of Laryngology, Rhinology, and Otology 1896;10(5):231–2.
36. Raw N. Foreign body in the oesophagus: localisation by X rays: successful removal. Br Med J 1896;2(1875):1678.
37. Fishman AJ, Roland JT Jr, Alexiades G, et al. Fluoroscopically assisted cochlear implantation. Otol Neurotol 2003;24(6):882–6.
38. Coelho DH, Waltzman SB, Roland JT Jr. Implanting common cavity malformations using intraoperative fluoroscopy. Otol Neurotol 2008;29(7):914–9.

39. Appachi S, Schwartz S, Ishman S, et al. Utility of intraoperative imaging in cochlear implantation: a systematic review. Laryngoscope 2018;128(8):1914–21.

40. Pieper S, Lorensen B, Schroeder W, et al. The NA-MIC Kit: ITK, VTK, pipelines, grids and 3D slicer as an open platform for the medical image computing community. Paper presented at: 3rd IEEE International Symposium on Biomedical Imaging: Nano to Macro. Arlington, VA, USA, April 6–9, 2006.

41. Johnson H, Harris G, Williams K. BRAINSFIT: mutual information registrations of whole-brain 3D Images, using the insight toolkit. Insight J 2007. http://hdl.handle.net/1926/1291. Accessed October 8, 2019.

42. Dees G, van Hoof M, Stokroos R. A proposed method for accurate 3D analysis of cochlear implant migration using fusion of cone beam CT. Front Surg 2016;3:2.

43. Curthoys IS, Markham CH, Curthoys EJ. Semicircular duct and ampulla dimensions in cat, guinea pig and man. J Morphol 1977;151(1):17–34.

44. van den Boogert T, van Hoof M, Handschuh S, et al. Optimization of 3D-visualization of micro-anatomical structures of the human inner ear in osmium tetroxide contrast enhanced micro-CT scans. Front Neuroanat 2018;12:41.

Vagal Nerve Stimulation
Indications, Implantation, and Outcomes

Kwaku K. Ohemeng, BS, Kourosh Parham, MD, PhD*

KEYWORDS

- Vagal nerve stimulation • VNS • Vagus nerve • Epilepsy • Seizure • Intractable
- Depression • Treatment resistant

KEY POINTS

- Vagal nerve stimulation (VNS) is indicated for treatment-resistant epilepsy and treatment-resistant depression and was approved by Food and Drug Administration for each of them in 1997 and 2005, respectively.
- The exact mechanism by which VNS achieves its effects is not known, but there are various proposed mechanisms such as increasing blood flow and neural activity in the brain.
- Outcomes of VNS include improvements in mood and effect and in daytime alertness/vigilance, reduction in the number of needed antiepileptic drugs, and improved behavioral outcomes in children.
- Commonly reported complications of VNS include hoarseness, throat pain/dysphagia, coughing, and shortness of breath; and most of these can be reduced by lowering the stimulation pulse width/frequency.

INTRODUCTION, RELEVANT ANATOMY, AND PHYSIOLOGY

The vagus nerve is the tenth cranial nerve (CN X). The name vagus is the Latin word meaning wandering,[1] which is fitting because it has the longest anatomic course of all the cranial nerves running from the medulla down into the abdomen. It is a major component of the autonomic nervous system (ANS) and plays an important role in regulating metabolic homeostasis.[2] The vagus nerve is a mixed nerve composed of about 80% afferent and about 20% efferent fibers.

The parasympathetic efferents of the vagus nerve arise from the dorsal nucleus of the vagus nerve in the brainstem.[3] They supply most of the organs below the neck as far as the left colonic (splenic) flexure[4]; these fibers constitute the main parasympathetic component of the ANS. The afferent sensory fibers of the vagus nerve relay taste information and visceral sensory information from the head and neck, thoracic,

Department of Surgery, Division of Otolaryngology–Head and Neck Surgery, UCONN School of Medicine, UConn Health, 263 Farmington Avenue, Farmington, CT 06030-8083, USA
* Corresponding author.
E-mail address: parham@uchc.edu

Otolaryngol Clin N Am 53 (2020) 127–143
https://doi.org/10.1016/j.otc.2019.09.008
0030-6665/20/© 2019 Elsevier Inc. All rights reserved.
oto.theclinics.com

and abdominal visceral organs[5] to the solitary tract nucleus in the brainstem. Together, these afferent and efferent pathways allow the vagus nerve to play its key role in the neuroendocrine-immune axis of maintaining homeostasis.[2] The vagus nerve also carries somatic afferent information from the mucosa of the larynx, posterior pinna, external auditory canal, and tympanic membrane to the spinal tract and spinal trigeminal nucleus in the brainstem.[4] Despite sensory information from both areas ultimately arriving at the same brainstem nucleus, it must be noted that the laryngeal mucosa above the glottis is innervated by the superior laryngeal nerve, whereas that below the glottis is innervated by the recurrent laryngeal nerve. This distinction is important clinically, as vagal nerve stimulation (VNS) implants are placed below the superior laryngeal branch of the vagus, and therefore its region of innervation is less likely to be affected by stimulation. In addition, the placement of VNS devices in this region of the vagus nerve is ideal as there are no other nerve branches there.[6] Overall, the brainstem (nuclei) distribution of the afferent vagal nerve fibers is important because presumably, it is the retrograde/anterograde stimulation of these fibers that endow the benefits of VNS therapy.[7]

The motor efferents of the vagus nerve arise from the nucleus ambiguus in the brainstem.[3] They control various skeletal muscles of the head and neck. This includes those involved in swallowing such as levator veli palatini; salpingopharyngeus; palatoglossus; palatopharyngeus; and the superior, middle, and inferior pharyngeal constrictor muscles.[8] The vagal nerve motor efferents also innervate the intrinsic muscles of larynx, which are primarily responsible for controlling vocal sound production by manipulation of the vocal folds. This includes the cricothyroid muscle (innervated by the superior laryngeal branch of the vagus), the lateral and posterior cricoarytenoid muscles, the thyroarytenoid muscles, the transverse and oblique arytenoid muscles, and the vocalis muscles (all of which are innervated by the recurrent laryngeal nerve branch of the vagus).[9] Therefore, any damage to the recurrent laryngeal nerve during surgical procedures can result in vocal cord paralysis, hoarseness, or other voice-related sequelae.

Although commonly referred to in the singular, the vagus nerve is a paired nerve consisting of a left and right vagus nerves. The left and right vagus nerves originate and develop symmetrically initially, but end up innervating different structures and therefore carry different kinds of information as the abdominal and thoracic organs rotate into their adult positions.[5] A clinically significant anatomic difference is right versus left vagal cardiac innervation: the right vagus nerve innervates the atria and along with the right sympathetic nerves affects the sinoatrial (SA) node more than the atrioventricular (AV) node, whereas the left vagus nerve innervates the ventricles and along with the left sympathetic nerves has more influence on the AV node than the SA node.[7,10] In addition, the density of innervation of the ventricles is less than that of the atria. Therefore, stimulation of the left vagal nerve is less likely to cause cardiac effects.[5,11,12] For this reason, VNS device implantation procedures are typically performed on the left vagal nerve. It must be noted, however, that significant overlap exists in the distribution of the neural input to the SA node and AV node,[7,10] and there have been reports of cardiac asystole due to VNS therapy[7,13,14] (see later section "Complications").

HISTORICAL BACKGROUND AND INDICATIONS FOR VAGAL NERVE STIMULATOR IMPLANTATION SURGERY

VNS refers to any technique that stimulates the vagus nerve, including manual or electrical stimulation.[2] In the 1880s, it was observed that the manual massage and compression of the carotid artery in the cervical region of the neck was able to mitigate seizure activity; this finding was attributed to stimulating the vagus nerve.[15] Subsequently, in the 1930s and 1940s, electrical VNS studies were performed on various animals to better understand its effects. It was found that VNS influenced brain electrical activity and that VNS had anticonvulsant effects.[2,16] From there, as early as the late 1980s, VNS was used successfully in humans to prevent intractable partial seizures.[17,18]

Between 1988 and 1998, five of the largest dedicated clinical trials of VNS for treating epilepsy called the E01-E05 trials were carried out. As a whole, these studies allowed for the performance of an open-label, long-term efficacy, safety, and tolerability study of VNS in a total of 454 patients with refractory epilepsy.[19] Various parameters of the enrolled patients including seizure frequency, medication treatment, and adverse events were measured at 6-month intervals and analyzed. It was found that long-term VNS therapy could achieve greater than or equal to 50% seizure reduction in 36.8% of patients at 1 year, 43.2% at 2 years, and in 42.7% at 3 years. VNS therapy also achieved median seizure reductions compared with baseline of 35% of patients at 1 year, 44.3% at 2 years, and 44.1% at 3 years.[19] These findings all occurred with VNS remaining safe and well-tolerated and having nearly 75% of patients choosing to continue therapy.[19]

The clear-cut findings of these trials eventually lead to the US Food and Drug Administration (FDA) approving the implantation of a VNS device for treating refractory epilepsy in 1997.[2,20] The approval specifically indicates the VNS therapy system for use as an adjunctive therapy in reducing the frequency of seizures in patients 4 years of age and older with partial onset seizures that are refractory to antiepileptic medications.[21]

Later, a 2000 study by Elger and colleagues[18] were the first to demonstrate VNS therapy causing an improvement in mood and affecting symptoms of patients with epilepsy that was independent of whether or not their seizures improved.[22] Since 2005, nearly 3000 clinical and preclinical VNS therapy papers have been published, with many focused on its use in epilepsy[18]; hence, VNS has been quite thoroughly studied in the context of epilepsy and to date, has remained a safe and tolerable adjunctive therapy option in refractory cases of epilepsy.

With regard to treating depression, the main rationale for using VNS therapy was initially based on and supported by various preclinical and clinical studies from the late 1990s and early 2000s.[2,23] Examples include the previously mentioned study by Elger and colleagues,[22] which demonstrated VNS having positive effects on mood and affecting symptoms of epileptic patients, even among patients whose seizures did not improve[2]; 1998 to 1999 studies by Harden and colleagues[24,25] in which PET imaging demonstrated evidence that VNS therapy directly affects the function of specific limbic structures of the brain[23]; neurochemical studies in animals and humans that demonstrated that VNS affects concentrations of monoamines (such as serotonin,[26] norepinephrine,[27] gamma-aminobutyric acid (GABA), and glutamate[28]) in the CNS[23]; and a 2004 study by Krahl, and colleagues[29] in which VNS was found to be an effective antidepressant in a rat model.

In 1998, the first open, unblinded 4-center study of VNS for the treatment of chronic or recurrent treatment-resistant depression (called D01) began.[23] It involved selecting patients with treatment-resistant, chronic, or recurrent major depressive episode (MDE) (unipolar or nonrapid cycling bipolar) and then adding VNS to a stable regiment of antidepressant medication or no antidepressant medications.[23] It showed some efficacy in very treatment-resistant patients, of whom 30.5% met the criteria for response after 3 months of VNS therapy[30,31] and interestingly, was more effective in depressed patients with lower degrees of treatment resistance.[23] Because the D01 study had the major shortcoming of exploring VNS effectiveness without using a controlled design, its interpretations of clinical utility were limited[30]; therefore further clinical trial investigation of VNS therapy for depression was necessary.

This subsequently led to the D02 study, which was a sham-controlled, multisite, double-blind trial with a larger sample size than the D01 study.[30] The D02 study did not demonstrate superiority of VNS therapy compared with sham treatment after 3 months,[30,32] but the longer-term (1 year) outcomes showed superior response rates in the D02 group patients when compared with patients from another observational study (the D04 study) who were a randomized, cluster-matched VNS-naïve treatment-resistant major depression episode population receiving "treatment as usual" (TAU).[30,33] The response rates were 27% in the D02 group compared with 13% in the D04 group, suggesting that VNS in addition to TAU was associated with a greater antidepressant benefit over 12 months.[34] Overall, these outcomes eventually led to the FDA approving Cyberonics VNS devices for treating chronic treatment-resistant major depressive disorder (TR-MDD) in 2005.[2,35] The approval was specifically for patients aged 18 years and older with treatment-resistant depression who failed to respond to at least 4 courses of adequate medication or electroconvulsive therapy (ECT).[33] Furthermore, various studies including a 5-year observational study from 2017 have demonstrated the efficacy of VNS in treating chronic TR-MDD and improving associated mortality outcomes.[36]

Despite these outcomes and prior FDA approval, the Centers for Medicare & Medicaid Services (CMS), the federal agency responsible for paying for much of US health care, withdrew their national coverage of VNS as an option for the treatment of TR-MDD in 2007.[37] This was because at the time, CMS determined that there was sufficient evidence that VNS was not reasonable and necessary for the treatment of resistant depression.[37] Regardless of this decision, it must be noted that any Medicare patients who were implanted with VNS devices between 2005 and 2007 are still covered by CMS and therefore eligible to have the pulse generator component replaced when its battery life runs out. In late 2018, there was a proposal to reestablish CMS coverage of VNS for treatment-resistant depression,[38] and furthermore, as of February 2019, the latest decision of the CMS is to support VNS implantation when offered in a CMS-approved, double-blind, randomized, placebo-controlled trial with a follow-up duration of at least 1 year.[39] CMS may extend to a prospective longitudinal study when the initial trials complete enrollment and if they have positive interim primary endpoint findings.[39]

Other non-FDA–approved uses of VNS, which have been explored in various case series reports and small open-label studies include rapid cycling bipolar disorder, treatment-resistant anxiety disorders, Alzheimer disease, chronic refractory headaches, and obesity.[2]

MECHANISM OF VAGAL NERVE STIMULATION

The exact mechanism of action by which VNS achieves seizure reduction is not known.[40] However, it is known that the mechanism is different from that of antiepileptic drugs that have direct effects on neuronal membrane ionic conductance or on neurotransmitter and receptor binding-site functions.[5,41] Various mechanisms have been suggested and are partially supported by animal and human studies, including, but not limited to the following:

1. Afferent vagal projections through the pontine parabrachial nucleus and thalamus to seizure-generating regions in the basal forebrain and insular cortex.[42] This

mechanism was suggested by a 1987 study by D.F. Cechetto and C.B. Saper in which they investigated the functional organization of the insular cortex of rats by recording neuronal responses to visceral sensory stimuli. Their results demonstrated that general and special visceral afferents to the insular cortex are organized in a viscerotopic manner. From this organization, they also found that afferent sensory information carried in the vagus nerve reached the cerebral cortex by a pathway involving the aforementioned regions (specifically the parabrachial nucleus of the dorsolateral pons and the ventroposterolateral parvicellular nucleus of the thalamus) and ended in the posterior granular insular cortex.[42]

2. Desynchronization of hypersynchronized cortical activity (ie, seizure activity) that depends on stimulus frequency and the strength of the electrical current.[43–45] This mechanism was suggested by a 1966 study by Chase and colleagues[43] in which they studied the cortical and subcortical activity patterns in the brains of cats after electrical stimulation of their cervical vagal nerves. They found that said stimulation was capable of eliciting both synchronized and desynchronized patterns of activity from the cerebral cortex and certain subcortical structures and that the given patterns that occurred depended on the specific parameters of the stimulation that was used.[43] The application of a given stimulus to evoke desynchronization in a given region of the cortex experiencing a seizure (ie, hypersynchronization) could potentially mitigate or even eliminate the given seizure.

3. Increased blood flow and neural activity in the thalamus, limbic system, and multiple cortical regions.[46] This mechanism was suggested by a 1992 study by Garnett and colleagues[46] in which they studied the regional cerebral blood flow (rCBF) in 5 patients who had received VNS implants for treatment of intractable seizures. They found specific rCBF changes localized to the anterior thalamus and anterior cingulate gyrus (both ipsilateral to the VNS implant). They also noted that the direct electrical stimulation of the anterior thalamus evoked metabolic responses in the limbic striate system.

4. Cortical inhibition secondary to release of inhibitory neurotransmitters, such as glycine and GABA.[47] This mechanism was suggested by a 2003 study by Marrosu and colleagues in which they used single-photon emission computed tomography to examine cortical $GABA_A$ receptor density (GRD) before and 1 year after implantation of a VNS device in 10 subjects with drug-resistant partial epilepsy. They found that VNS therapeutic responses significantly correlated with the normalization of GRD and that a comparable control group that only took antiepileptic medication for 1 year (without VNS therapy) failed to show significant GRD variations.[47]

SURGICAL IMPLANTATION PROCEDURE

A commonly used standard VNS device is a commercially available programmable pulse generator device (namely the neurocybernetic prosthesis system), which was developed by Cyberonics Inc. (Houston, TX, USA) for the treatment of human epilepsy.[2,5] Its components include the following: a pulse generator, a bipolar VNS lead, a programming wand with accompanying computer software, a tunneling tool, and hand-held magnets.[5] To properly implant a given VNS device, the stimulating electrodes must be put in direct contact with the vagus nerve itself (**Fig. 1**). This allows for the transportation of the electrical signal from the pulse generator to the vagus nerve. Electrode coils are helical to easily wrap around the vagus nerve without causing trauma as well as maximize contact surface area with the nerve itself.[5] The procedure is about 1 to 1.5 hours long and is typically done under general anesthesia to minimize seizures or the occurrence of events that may compromise the surgery.[5]

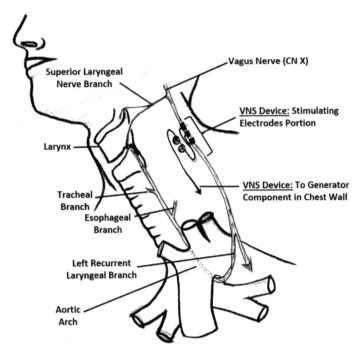

Fig. 1. The left vagus (CN X) nerve with laryngeal branches and VNS leads in place below the superior laryngeal nerve branching point.

First, the vagus nerve itself is exposed in a manner similar to a carotid endarterectomy procedure. An incision is made over the anterior border of the left sternocleidomastoid muscle, centered between the mastoid process and clavicle. This particular region on the vagus nerve is between the superior and inferior cervical cardiac branches and above the left recurrent laryngeal nerve. It is the recommended stimulation site, as the vagus nerve is usually clear of branches there.[6]

The vagus nerve is typically identified within a posterior groove in the carotid sheath between the carotid artery and the internal jugular vein. Vessel loops can then be used to mobilize the vagus nerve to allow for a minimum of 3 cm exposure for the attachment of the helical coils.[5] Excessive handling and drying out of the nerve should be avoided during surgery; these can result in nerve damage and/or swelling and the patient may clinically present with postoperative vocal cord paralysis.[6] Next, another incision must be made for the placement of the pulse generator component of the VNS device. This incision is made about 8 cm inferior to the left clavicle and is centered under the midpoint of the clavicle. A subcutaneous pouch is made above the incision or along the axillary border for the placement of the generator and excess lead.[5,6] The tunneling tool component is then used to move the ends of the electrodes from the base of the cervical incision to the thoracic incision. The helical coils are then carefully wrapped around the exposed vagus nerve. Then the pulse generator is brought into the surgical fields and attached to the electrode connector pins.[5]

Before placing the pulse generator in the subcutaneous pouch and closing incisions, the diagnostic testing and device interrogation must be done to ensure the VNS system is functioning properly. The system diagnostic testing evaluates the lead impedance of the VNS system and the pulse generator's ability to successfully deliver the programmed stimulation.[6] Interrogation is done to ensure proper device communication between the programming wand and the implanted system. Typically 2 diagnostic tests are performed: the first one out of pocket to verify connection and the second one in pocket to verify if the VNS implant depth is adequate. The anesthesiologist is informed of the potential risk of bradycardia or asystole before diagnostics are run. Similar to diagnostic testing, interrogation should be done twice: first outside of the sterile field while still in the sterile package and second when the generator is placed in the pocket and before the skin is closed. Interrogation should verify that normal mode and magnet mode outputs are both 0.0 mA.[6] Successful communication is most likely if the programming wand is within 1 inch of the pulse generator.[6]

Lastly, both incision sites are irrigated before closure. Scarring is minimized using subcuticular closure for both skin incisions. At the physician's discretion postoperative antibiotics can be administered.[6] Postoperatively, neck and chest radiographs can be obtained to confirm the proper placement of the generator and electrodes.[5] It must be noted that the battery of the generator component is integrated and has a finite lifespan. Therefore, depending on the intensity and frequency of stimulation, the pulse generator will need to be replaced every 5 plus years. This is one of the reasons for revision surgery (discussed later). For this reason, the VNS lead is made such that it can be easily inserted and removed from the pulse generator. System diagnostics and device interrogation are performed in the same manner on pulse generator replacement as in initial device installation.

REVISION SURGERY PROCEDURE

The most common reason for revision surgery is pulse generator replacement.[6] This is usually due to the device battery running low; most devices have a threshold voltage, which if dropped below, an "End of Service" (EOS) flag is triggered. This nonzero threshold voltage allows for the replacement to be made before completely running out of battery. High impedance is another reason for revision surgery. Common causes of high impedance include lead breaks, improper connection between generator and lead pin, poor attachment of lead electrodes to the vagus nerve, fibrosis between the electrode and the vagus nerve, and generator malfunction.[6] High impedance can be corrected by lead pin reinsertion, lead replacement, generator replacement, or both lead and generator replacement. Other reasons for revision surgery may be adverse events such as infection, device extrusion, protrusion, or migration. These adverse events may require full or partial explant before reimplantation.[6]

As previously noted, system diagnostic testing and device interrogation should be performed before any revision or replacement surgery. This is important because the results will determine what aspects of the VNS device must be replaced. If communication cannot be established with the generator due to battery depletion, the integrity of the system (ie, status of lead) cannot be confirmed. In this situation, one should be prepared to perform a full system revision, if necessary. Radiographs should be taken, as they will be needed during the surgical revision case to confirm generator location, prevent cutting or nicking of the lead, and to verify that there are no lead breaks or discontinuities.[6]

The pulse generator replacement procedure is fairly straightforward: the existing generator is removed from the pocket (with the lead pin still connected); the new generator package is opened; the existing generator is disconnected from the implanted lead; and the replacement generator is connected to the leads. If the new generator is smaller than the previous one, there will be an extraneous pocket space left behind. If left alone, this pocket may increase the likelihood of certain adverse events (such as seroma development, device manipulation, and device migration).[6] The suture hole present on the VNS device should be used to fixate the device to fascia after installation to minimize adverse events.

The lead pin replacement is as follows: a neck incision is opened and the vagus nerve/helices interface is located; the degree of fibrotic encapsulation is then assessed to determine if the entire lead can be safely removed; if possible, the existing helices are removed and the new helices are placed in the same location; otherwise, the existing lead is transected leaving no more than 4 cm remaining; new leads are then connected to the existing generator; and diagnostic testing and final interrogation are then performed.[6] If too much fibrosis prevents safe removal of the leads, the lead wire is cut with the leads left in place. A new lead is then implanted immediately below the old leads.

OUTCOMES

With regard to nonseizure outcomes, one commonly reported is improvements in quality of life measures in both children and adults who undergo VNS therapy.[48,49] Although this is mostly secondary to reduction in seizures—as the effect is greatest in those who achieve the highest reduction in seizures—there is an effect that is independent of seizure reduction frequency and may be related to the effects of CNS on mood, alertness, and other factors.[40] Paralleling seizure reduction effects, improvement in quality of life measures tend to increase over time with VNS therapy.[40]

The effect of VNS therapy on mood symptoms is an outcome worth considering. Most of the evidence suggesting that VNS improves mood or other depressive symptoms in patients with epilepsy is inconclusive.[40,50] There are studies such as the previously mentioned 2000 study by G. Elger[22] and a similar 2001 study by C. Hoppe[51] that showed positive mood effects in patients receiving VNS for intractable seizure disorders. The latter study notes that the absolute reduction in seizures may contribute to the antidysphoric effect seen.[51] VNS is still currently being investigated as a treatment of depression in nonepileptic patients. Although some open-label and observational studies suggest that VNS may have some efficacy in treating depression,[36,40,52] it must be noted that a randomized control trial (the D02 study) did not find any benefit compared with sham stimulation over the initial 3-month period.[32] Despite this, it is possible that the benefit of VNS therapy for treatment-resistant depression builds up over time, based on the findings of prospective observational studies that observed patients for one or more years.[53,54]

Another outcome to consider with VNS is its effect on mortality rates. Compared with the expected rates in the intractable epilepsy population, patients receiving VNS therapy seem to have the same rates of overall mortality and/or sudden death.[40] However, it must be noted that there is evidence that VNS may reduce the rates of sudden unexplained death in epilepsy (SUDEP); specifically, in a cohort of 1819 individuals followed-up after VNS implantations, the SUDEP rate was about 5.5 per 100 over the first 2 years but only 1.7 per 1000 thereafter.[40,55]

VNS therapy can also improve daytime alertness/vigilance and reduce daytime sleepiness despite its potential to exacerbate sleep apnea.[3,40,56,57] The improved alertness was found to occur in some patients even without significant reduction in seizure frequency.[56] This effect may be due to the stimulation of vagal brainstem centers that promote alertness such as the parabrachial nucleus and locus ceruleus.[40]

Another nonseizure outcome found to be associated with VNS therapy is a reduction in the number of needed antiepileptic drugs and/or dosages[58]—in some cases patients become seizure free with VNS therapy and no drug treatment.[59,60]

Information regarding the frequency of this particular outcome is limited[40]: some larger studies suggest that most patients remain on the same number of antiepileptic drugs without discussing dosing alterations,[19,48,58] whereas various smaller case series report the contrary with more antiepileptic drug reductions.[60]

VNS has also been found to be associated with improved behavioral outcomes in children with autism and intellectual disability such as improved alertness, mental age, and performance on some functional measured and cognitive tests.[48,61,62]

COMPLICATIONS

Two of the five previously mentioned large VNS studies from the late 1990s—namely the E03 trial (conducted in 1995 by Vagus Nerve Stimulation Study Group)[63] and the E05 trial (conducted in 1998 by Handforth and colleagues[64])—provide good information regarding side effects experienced by patients receiving VNS therapy. The most commonly reported side effects of high ($\geq$2.25 mA) stimulation VNS from the E03 trial were hoarseness (37%), throat pain (11%), coughing (7%), shortness of breath (6%), tingling (6%), and muscle pain (6%). From the E05 trial, shortness of breath, pharyngitis, and voice alteration were reported (specifically more so with high-stimulation VNS than low [0.25–1.0 mA] stimulation).[40] Generally, reducing the pulse width of stimulation and/or the frequency can reduce the side effects related to VNS stimulation.[40,65] Implantation site infection, usually of the subcutaneous pocket containing the generator with *Staphylococcus aureus*, occurs in 2% to 7% of cases.[66] In such cases, systemic antibiotics, removal of the device, or open wound debridement is required.[40] Although physiologic studies have typically not found any clinically relevant effect of VNS therapy on cardiorespiratory function,[67,68] bradycardia followed by transient asystole lasting up to 45 seconds has been reported in approximately 0.1% of cases.[13,14,40,69] There is also a known case of VNS causing late-onset, periodic asystolic episodes resulting in syncopal events.[7]

An ENT-specific complication found to occur with VNS surgery is unilateral vocal cord paralysis, which occurs in about 1% of cases[40] and is directly attributable to intraoperative manipulation of the recurrent laryngeal nerve.[63,66] Although most of these patients recover,[40] there are at least 2 known cases of permanent vocal cord paralysis that occurred several weeks after implantation.[70] It must be noted that in these cases the damage was self-inflicted by patients who externally manipulated their VNS devices presumably placing traction on the recurrent laryngeal nerve.[70] There are some observations of VNS therapy inducing or worsening sleep apnea syndrome.[71,72] For those with preexisting sleep apnea, VNS was found to be associated with more frequent apnea and hypopnea episodes in sleep.[40] Lowering stimulus frequency was found to reduce VNS-related apnea and hypopnea,[73] whereas in other cases continuous positive airway pressure was needed.[72] Some other very rare side effects that have been reported in at least 1 case include the following: pneumothorax,[66] gastrointestinal side effects such as chronic diarrhea,[74] muscle spasms including uncomfortable chest wall spasms[75] and sternocleidomastoid contraction,[76] and other cranial nerve palsies such as Horner syndrome and facial paralysis.[77]

Important to also note are the symptoms commonly experienced by patients initially on activation of the implanted VNS system (ie, stimulation-induced symptoms and side effects). Generally, most stimulation-induced symptoms can be minimized by reducing stimulation intensity.[54] The most common are similar to the side effects previously discussed and include dysphonia (hoarseness), coughing, and dysphagia/throat pain. Per an analysis of the acute phase of the E03 VNS trial, these were found to occur in 35.5%, 13.9%, and 12.9% of patients, respectively.[78] Other stimulation-induced symptoms include neck pain, paresthesias, vomiting, dyspepsia, headaches, and hypomania or mania.[53] A 2003 study by Smyth and colleagues[79] that explored VNS therapy for children found various other stimulation-induced symptoms (in addition to dysphonia and dysphagia), such as cough, drooling, torticollis, outbursts of laughter, shoulder abduction, and urinary retention. Of those, excluding dysphonia and dysphagia, the most common was torticollis (occurring in 5.4% of cases).[79] Other specific symptoms have been noted to occur at higher stimulation currents, in particular, pain and/or discomfort especially in VNS-naïve patients receiving therapy who are not used to higher current outputs.[80,81] Many previously mentioned VNS side effects such as voice alteration, cough, feeling of throat tightening, and dyspnea are known to occur more often at higher currents.[80] More rare side effects found to be associated with VNS at high currents include cardiac side effects such as bradycardia and asystole.[81] A 1993 study by Lundy and colleagues[82] that focused primarily on laryngeal effects of VNS noted laryngeal hemi-spasm (laryngismus) with high stimulation. Two individual case reports (one adult case from 2000[83] and one pediatric case from 2018[84]) have noted the aggravation of preexisting seizures on increasing the VNS current output to relatively high levels (to 2.5 mA and 2.0 mA, respectively) after 3 to 4 months of therapy. The pediatric patient also experienced status epilepticus following the worsening seizures.[84] The complications of VNS therapy are summarized in **Table 1**.

CONTRAINDICATIONS

The main contraindication to VNS therapy is baseline cardiac conduction disorders. This is because there is the potential for efferent conduction through the vagus nerve, especially on the right, to worsen cardiac conduction abnormalities.[40] VNS therapy is also contraindicated in patients who have undergone bilateral or left cervical vagotomy procedures.[6] Diathermy, specifically shortwave, microwave, and therapeutic ultrasound diathermy are contraindicated in patients implanted with a VNS therapy system; but diagnostic ultrasound is not included in this contraindication.[6] This contraindication is because diathermy can cause heating of the VNS therapy system well above temperatures required for tissue destruction[33]; this

Table 1
Complications of vagal nerve stimulation therapy

Complication	Percentage of Cases
Hoarseness (dysphonia)	37%
Throat pain	11%
Coughing	7%
Shortness of breath (dyspnea)	6%
Tingling	6%
Muscle pain	6%
Implantation site infection	2%–7%
Unilateral vocal cord paralysis (temporary)	1%
Bradycardia + transient asystole	Rare (<1%)
Pneumothorax	Rare (<1%)
GI side effects (chronic diarrhea)	Rare (<1%)
Muscle spasms (chest wall, SCM muscle)	Rare (<1%)
Cranial nerve palsies (Horner syndrome, facial paralysis)	Rare (<1%)

Table 2
Contraindications to vagal nerve stimulation therapy

Contraindication	Type	Important Notes
Bilateral or left vagotomy Procedure previously undergone	Absolute	
Baseline cardiac conduction disorders	Absolute	
Diathermy (shortwave, microwave, therapeutic ultrasound)	Absolute	Diagnostic ultrasound is safe to use with the VNS therapy system
Sleep apnea	Relative	
MRI	Relative	The MRI usage protocol must be modified; MRI cannot be used in torso region containing the VNS therapy system
Programmable shunt valves	Relative	There are some reported cases of VNS magnets affecting shunts; VNS stimulation with magnet should be avoided

can furthermore cause damage that may result in pain or discomfort, loss of vocal cord function, or even possibly death if there is damage to blood vessels.[33] Sleep apnea is a relative contraindication for VNS therapy. This is based on aforementioned findings that VNS can induce or worsen sleep apnea syndrome.[71,72] Therefore, before VNS implantation surgery, patients should have possible sleep apnea–related symptoms and physical signs sought out on history and physical examination. If these symptoms are found, necessary testing should be pursued to determine if the patient has clinically significant sleep apnea.[40] There are also some specific cases of programmable shunt valves being affected by the use of VNS magnets.[85] VNS stimulation using the magnet should be avoided in patients with programmable shunts.[40] Despite the VNS system being an implanted metallic device, the usage of MRI is safe and allowed in VNS patients provided that specific guidelines or a modified MRI protocol is followed.[86] The modified MRI protocols used are device specific and require that the torso region containing the VNS therapy system (including the generator and lead) is not exposed to the radio frequency field of the MRI.[87,88] This region is typically between C7 and T8 (or in some cases C7 to L3); hence, the extremities and the head and neck can usually be safely scanned with MRI in VNS patients. Regardless, the providing physician should be contacted before getting an MRI to verify any device-specific safety measures to be considered beforehand. VNS therapy contraindications are summarized in **Table 2**.

SUMMARY

In summary, VNS therapy is a surgical treatment that involves the implantation of a device to electrically stimulate the left vagus nerve. Its main indications are the following: (1) for epilepsy, specifically as an adjunctive therapy in reducing the frequency of seizures in patients 4 years of age and older with partial onset seizures that are refractory to antiepileptic medications[21] and (2) for depression, specifically for patients aged 18 years and older with treatment-resistant depression who failed to respond to at least 4 courses of adequate medication or ECT.[33] VNS therapy is safe to use in any patients meeting these indications, excluding those with contraindications previously discussed. VNS patients can safely receive most forms of imaging including computed tomography, radiography, and ultrasound without restrictions and can receive MRI in any areas excluding the regions where the VNS system resides.[89]

DISCLOSURE

The authors have nothing to disclose.

REFERENCES

1. Lewis CT, văgus SC. A latin dictionary founded on Andrews' edition of Freund's latin dictionary. 1879. Available at: http://www.perseus.tufts.edu/hopper/text?doc=Perseus:text:1999.04.0059:entry=vagus. Accessed March 2, 2019.
2. Howland RH. Vagus nerve stimulation. Curr Behav Neurosci Rep 2014;1(2): 64–73.
3. Galli R, Bonanni E, Pizzanelli C, et al. Daytime vigilance and quality of life in epileptic patients treated with vagus nerve stimulation. Epilepsy Behav 2003; 4(2):185–91. Available at: http://www.ncbi.nlm.nih.gov/pubmed/12697145.
4. Tewfik TL. Vagus nerve anatomy. Medscape; 2017. Available at: https://emedicine.medscape.com/article/1875813-overview. Accessed March 3, 2019.
5. Schachter SC, Saper CB. Vagus nerve stimulation. Epilepsia 1998;39(7):677–86.
6. Cyberonics. VNS Therapy® system: surgical implant procedure and outcomes [CD-ROM] 2011.
7. Ratajczak T, Blank R, Parikh A, et al. Late-onset asystolic episodes in a patient with a vagal nerve stimulator. HeartRhythm Case Rep 2018;4(7):314–7.
8. Netter FH. Vagus nerve (X): schema. In: Hansen JT, Benninger B, Brueckner-Collins J, et al, editors. Atlas of human anatomy (netter basic science). 6th edition. Philadelphia: Elsevier/Saunders; 2014. p. 131.
9. Netter FH. Muscle tables. In: Hansen JT, Benninger B, Brueckner-Collins J, et al, editors. Atlas of human anatomy (netter basic science). 6th edition. Philadelphia: Elsevier/Saunders; 2014. p. 156–61.
10. Mann DL, Zipes DP, Libby P, et al. Braunwald's heart disease: a textbook of cardiovascular medicine. 10th edition. Philadelphia: Elsevier/Saunders; 2014.
11. Stemper B, Devinsky O, Haendl T, et al. Effects of vagus nerve stimulation on cardiovascular regulation in patients with epilepsy. Acta Neurol Scand 2008;117(4): 231–6.
12. Sperling W, Reulbach U, Bleich S, et al. Cardiac effects of vagus nerve stimulation in patients with major depression. Pharmacopsychiatry 2010;43(01):7–11.
13. Schuurman PR, Beukers RJ. Ventricular asystole during vagal nerve stimulation. Epilepsia 2009;50(4):967–8.
14. Tatum WO, Moore DB, Stecker MM, et al. Ventricular asystole during vagus nerve stimulation for epilepsy in humans. Neurology 1999;52(6):1267.
15. Lanska DJ. J.L. Corning and vagal nerve stimulation for seizures in the 1880s. Neurology 2002;58(3):452–9. Available at: http://www.ncbi.nlm.nih.gov/pubmed/11839848.
16. Zabara J. Inhibition of experimental seizures in canines by repetitive vagal stimulation. Epilepsia 1992;33(6):1005–12. Available at: http://www.ncbi.nlm.nih.gov/pubmed/1464256.
17. Penry JK, Dean JC. Prevention of intractable partial seizures by intermittent vagal stimulation in humans: preliminary results. Epilepsia 1990;31(Suppl 2):S40–3. Available at: http://www.ncbi.nlm.nih.gov/pubmed/2121469.

18. Carreno FR, Frazer A. Vagal nerve stimulation for treatment-resistant depression. Neurotherapeutics 2017;14(3):716–27.
19. Morris GL, Mueller WM. Long-term treatment with vagus nerve stimulation in patients with refractory epilepsy. The Vagus Nerve Stimulation Study Group E01-E05. Neurology 1999;53(8):1731–5. Available at: http://www.ncbi.nlm.nih.gov/pubmed/10563620.
20. Morris GL, Gloss D, Buchhalter J, et al. Evidence-based guideline update: Vagus nerve stimulation for the treatment of epilepsy: Report of the Guideline Development Subcommittee of the American Academy of Neurology. Neurology 2013; 81(16):1453–9.
21. Center for Devices and Radiological Health (CDRH). Summary of Safety and Effectiveness Data - VNS TherapyTM System (Epilepsy) [PDF file]. Food and Drug Administration (FDA) Website. 2017. Available at: https://www.accessdata.fda.gov/cdrh_docs/pdf/p970003s207b.pdf. Accessed March 16, 2019.
22. Elger G, Hoppe C, Falkai P, et al. Vagus nerve stimulation is associated with mood improvements in epilepsy patients. Epilepsy Res 2000;42(2–3):203–10. Available at: http://www.ncbi.nlm.nih.gov/pubmed/11074193.
23. George MS, Rush AJ, Sackeim HA, et al. Vagus nerve stimulation (VNS): utility in neuropsychiatric disorders. Int J Neuropsychopharmacol 2003;6(1). S1461145703003250.
24. Henry TR, Bakay RA, Votaw JR, et al. Brain blood flow alterations induced by therapeutic vagus nerve stimulation in partial epilepsy: I. Acute effects at high and low levels of stimulation. Epilepsia 1998;39(9):983–90. Available at: http://www.ncbi.nlm.nih.gov/pubmed/9738678.
25. Henry TR, Votaw JR, Pennell PB, et al. Acute blood flow changes and efficacy of vagus nerve stimulation in partial epilepsy. Neurology 1999;52(6):1166–73. Available at: http://www.ncbi.nlm.nih.gov/pubmed/10214738.
26. Ben-Menachem E, Hamberger A, Hedner T, et al. Effects of vagus nerve stimulation on amino acids and other metabolites in the CSF of patients with partial seizures. Epilepsy Res 1995;20(3):221–7. Available at: http://www.ncbi.nlm.nih.gov/pubmed/7796794.
27. Krahl SE, Clark KB, Smith DC, et al. Locus coeruleus lesions suppress the seizure-attenuating effects of vagus nerve stimulation. Epilepsia 1998;39(7): 709–14. Available at: http://www.ncbi.nlm.nih.gov/pubmed/9670898.
28. Walker BR, Easton A, Gale K. Regulation of limbic motor seizures by GABA and glutamate transmission in nucleus tractus solitarius. Epilepsia 1999;40(8): 1051–7. Available at: http://www.ncbi.nlm.nih.gov/pubmed/10448815.
29. Krahl SE, Senanayake SS, Pekary AE, et al. Vagus nerve stimulation (VNS) is effective in a rat model of antidepressant action. J Psychiatr Res 2004;38(3): 237–40.
30. Schlaepfer TE, Frick C, Zobel A, et al. Vagus nerve stimulation for depression: efficacy and safety in a European study. Psychol Med 2008;38(05). https://doi.org/10.1017/S0033291707001924.
31. Rush AJ, George MS, Sackeim HA, et al. Vagus nerve stimulation (VNS) for treatment-resistant depressions: a multicenter study. Biol Psychiatry 2000;47(4): 276–86. Available at: http://www.ncbi.nlm.nih.gov/pubmed/10686262.
32. Rush AJ, Marangell LB, Sackeim HA, et al. Vagus nerve stimulation for treatment-resistant depression: a randomized, controlled acute phase trial. Biol Psychiatry 2005;58(5):347–54.

33. Center for Devices and Radiological Health (CDRH). Summary of Safety and Effectiveness Data - VNS Therapy™ System (Depression) [PDF file]. Food and Drug Administration (FDA) Website. 2005. Available at: www.accessdata.fda.gov/cdrh_docs/pdf/P970003S050b.pdf. Accessed March 15, 2019.

34. Eljamel S. Vagus nerve stimulation for major depressive episodes. Prog Neurol Surg 2015;53–63. https://doi.org/10.1159/000434655.

35. Howland RH, Shutt LS, Berman SR, et al. The emerging use of technology for the treatment of depression and other neuropsychiatric disorders. Ann Clin Psychiatry 2011;23(1):48–62. Available at: http://www.ncbi.nlm.nih.gov/pubmed/21318196.

36. Aaronson ST, Sears P, Ruvuna F, et al. A 5-year observational study of patients with treatment-resistant depression treated with vagus nerve stimulation or treatment as usual: comparison of response, remission, and suicidality. Am J Psychiatry 2017;174(7):640–8.

37. Centers for Medicare & Medicaid Services (CMS). Decision Memo for Vagus Nerve Stimulation for Treatment of Resistant Depression (TRD) (CAG-00313R). Centers for Medicare & Medicaid Services Website. 2007. Available at: https://www.cms.gov/medicare-coverage-database/details/nca-decision-memo.aspx?NCAId=195. Accessed March 26, 2019.

38. Centers for Medicare & Medicaid Services (CMS). Proposed Decision Memo for Vagus Nerve Stimulation (VNS) for Treatment Resistant Depression (TRD) (CAG-00313R2). Centers for Medicare & Medicaid Services Website. 2018. Available at: https://www.cms.gov/medicare-coverage-database/details/nca-proposed-decision-memo.aspx?NCAId=292. Accessed March 26, 2019.

39. Centers for Medicare & Medicaid Services (CMS). Decision Memo for Vagus Nerve Stimulation (VNS) for Treatment Resistant Depression (TRD) (CAG-00313R2). Centers for Medicare & Medicaid Services Website. 2019. Available at: https://www.cms.gov/medicare-coverage-database/details/nca-decision-memo.aspx?NCAId=292. Accessed March 26, 2019.

40. Schachter SC. Vagus nerve stimulation therapy for the treatment of epilepsy. UpToDate; 2018. Available at: https://www.uptodate.com/contents/vagus-nerve-stimulation-therapy-for-the-treatment-of-epilepsy. Accessed March 3, 2019.

41. Davies JA. Mechanisms of action of antiepileptic drugs. Seizure 1995;4(4):267–71. Available at: http://www.ncbi.nlm.nih.gov/pubmed/8719918.

42. Cechetto DF, Saper CB. Evidence for a viscerotopic sensory representation in the cortex and thalamus in the rat. J Comp Neurol 1987;262(1):27–45.

43. Chase MH, Sterman MB, Clemente CD. Cortical and subcortical patterns of response to afferent vagal stimulation. Exp Neurol 1966;16(1):36–49. Available at: http://www.ncbi.nlm.nih.gov/pubmed/5923482.

44. Chase MH, Nakamura Y, Clemente CD, et al. Afferent vagal stimulation: neurographic correlates of induced EEG synchronization and desynchronization. Brain Res 1967;5(2):236–49. Available at: http://www.ncbi.nlm.nih.gov/pubmed/6033149.

45. Chase MH, Nakamura Y. Cortical and subcortical EEG patterns of response to afferent abdominal vagal stimulation: Neurographic correlates. Physiol Behav 1968;3(5):605–10.

46. Garnett ES, Nahmias C, Scheffel A, et al. Regional cerebral blood flow in man manipulated by direct vagal stimulation. Pacing Clin Electrophysiol 1992;15(10 Pt 2):1579–80. Available at: http://www.ncbi.nlm.nih.gov/pubmed/1383972.

47. Di Lazzaro V, Oliviero A, Pilato F, et al. Effects of vagus nerve stimulation on cortical excitability in epileptic patients. Neurology 2004;62(12):2310–2. Available at: http://www.ncbi.nlm.nih.gov/pubmed/15210904.

48. Murphy JV, Torkelson R, Dowler I, et al. Vagal nerve stimulation in refractory epilepsy: the first 100 patients receiving vagal nerve stimulation at a pediatric epilepsy center. Arch Pediatr Adolesc Med 2003;157(6):560–4.

49. Patwardhan RV, Stong B, Bebin EM, et al. Efficacy of vagal nerve stimulation in children with medically refractory epilepsy. Neurosurgery 2000;47(6): 1353–7 [discussion: 1357–8]. Available at: http://www.ncbi.nlm.nih.gov/pubmed/11126906.

50. Harden CL, Pulver MC, Ravdin LD, et al. A pilot study of mood in epilepsy patients treated with vagus nerve stimulation. Epilepsy Behav 2000;1(2):93–9.

51. Hoppe C, Helmstaedter C, Scherrmann J, et al. Self-reported mood changes following 6 months of vagus nerve stimulation in epilepsy patients. Epilepsy Behav 2001;2(4):335–42.

52. Rush AJ, Sackeim HA, Marangell LB, et al. Effects of 12 months of vagus nerve stimulation in treatment-resistant depression: a naturalistic study. Biol Psychiatry 2005;58(5):355–63.

53. Holtzheimer PE. Unipolar depression in adults: treatment with surgical approaches. UpToDate; 2017. Available at: https://www.uptodate.com/contents/unipolar-depression-in-adults-treatment-with-surgical-approaches. Accessed March 15, 2019.

54. Kennedy SH, Milev R, Giacobbe P, et al. Canadian Network for Mood and Anxiety Treatments (CANMAT) Clinical guidelines for the management of major depressive disorder in adults. IV. Neurostimulation therapies. J Affect Disord 2009; 117(Suppl):S44–53.

55. Annegers JF, Coan SP, Hauser WA, et al. Epilepsy, vagal nerve stimulation by the NCP system, all-cause mortality, and sudden, unexpected, unexplained death. Epilepsia 2000;41(5):549–53. Available at: http://www.ncbi.nlm.nih.gov/pubmed/10802760.

56. Malow BA, Edwards J, Marzec M, et al. Vagus nerve stimulation reduces daytime sleepiness in epilepsy patients. Neurology 2001;57(5):879–84. Available at: http://www.ncbi.nlm.nih.gov/pubmed/11552020.

57. Frost M, Gates J, Helmers SL, et al. Vagus nerve stimulation in children with refractory seizures associated with Lennox-Gastaut syndrome. Epilepsia 2001; 42(9):1148–52. Available at: http://www.ncbi.nlm.nih.gov/pubmed/11580762.

58. Labar DR. Antiepileptic drug use during the first 12 months of vagus nerve stimulation therapy: a registry study. Neurology 2002;59(6 Suppl 4):S38–43. Available at: http://www.ncbi.nlm.nih.gov/pubmed/12270967.

59. Labar D, Murphy J, Tecoma E. Vagus nerve stimulation for medication-resistant generalized epilepsy. E04 VNS Study Group. Neurology 1999;52(7):1510–2. Available at: http://www.ncbi.nlm.nih.gov/pubmed/10227649.

60. Tatum WO, Johnson KD, Goff S, et al. Vagus nerve stimulation and drug reduction. Neurology 2001;56(4):561–3. Available at: http://www.ncbi.nlm.nih.gov/pubmed/11261422.

61. Parker AP, Polkey CE, Binnie CD, et al. Vagal nerve stimulation in epileptic encephalopathies. Pediatrics 1999;103(4 Pt 1):778–82. Available at: http://www.ncbi.nlm.nih.gov/pubmed/10103302.

62. Aldenkamp AP, Van de Veerdonk SH, Majoie HJ, et al. Effects of 6 months of treatment with vagus nerve stimulation on behavior in children with lennox-gastaut

syndrome in an open clinical and nonrandomized study. Epilepsy Behav 2001; 2(4):343–50.

63. A randomized controlled trial of chronic vagus nerve stimulation for treatment of medically intractable seizures. The Vagus Nerve Stimulation Study Group. Neurology 1995;45(2):224–30. Available at: http://www.ncbi.nlm.nih.gov/pubmed/7854516.

64. Handforth A, DeGiorgio CM, Schachter SC, et al. Vagus nerve stimulation therapy for partial-onset seizures: a randomized active-control trial. Neurology 1998; 51(1):48–55. Available at: http://www.ncbi.nlm.nih.gov/pubmed/9674777.

65. Liporace J, Hucko D, Morrow R, et al. Vagal nerve stimulation: adjustments to reduce painful side effects. Neurology 2001;57(5):885–6. Available at: http://www.ncbi.nlm.nih.gov/pubmed/11552021.

66. Elliott RE, Morsi A, Kalhorn SP, et al. Vagus nerve stimulation in 436 consecutive patients with treatment-resistant epilepsy: long-term outcomes and predictors of response. Epilepsy Behav 2011;20(1):57–63.

67. Frei MG, Osorio I. Left vagus nerve stimulation with the neurocybernetic prosthesis has complex effects on heart rate and on its variability in humans. Epilepsia 2001;42(8):1007–16. Available at: http://www.ncbi.nlm.nih.gov/pubmed/11554886.

68. Binks AP, Paydarfar D, Schachter SC, et al. High strength stimulation of the vagus nerve in awake humans: a lack of cardiorespiratory effects. Respir Physiol 2001; 127(2–3):125–33. Available at: http://www.ncbi.nlm.nih.gov/pubmed/11504585.

69. Asconapé JJ, Moore DD, Zipes DP, et al. Bradycardia and asystole with the use of vagus nerve stimulation for the treatment of epilepsy: a rare complication of intraoperative device testing. Epilepsia 1999;40(10):1452–4. Available at: http://www.ncbi.nlm.nih.gov/pubmed/10528943.

70. Kalkanis JG, Krishna P, Espinosa JA, et al. Self-inflicted vocal cord paralysis in patients with vagus nerve stimulators. Report of two cases. J Neurosurg 2002; 96(5):949–51.

71. Holmes MD, Chang M, Kapur V. Sleep apnea and excessive daytime somnolence induced by vagal nerve stimulation. Neurology 2003;61(8):1126–9. Available at: http://www.ncbi.nlm.nih.gov/pubmed/14581678.

72. Marzec M, Edwards J, Sagher O, et al. Effects of vagus nerve stimulation on sleep-related breathing in epilepsy patients. Epilepsia 2003;44(7):930–5. Available at: http://www.ncbi.nlm.nih.gov/pubmed/12823576.

73. Malow BA, Edwards J, Marzec M, et al. Effects of vagus nerve stimulation on respiration during sleep: a pilot study. Neurology 2000;55(10):1450–4. Available at: http://www.ncbi.nlm.nih.gov/pubmed/11094096.

74. Sanossian N, Haut S. Chronic diarrhea associated with vagal nerve stimulation. Neurology 2002;58(2):330. Available at: http://www.ncbi.nlm.nih.gov/pubmed/11805274.

75. Leijten FS, Van Rijen PC. Stimulation of the phrenic nerve as a complication of vagus nerve pacing in a patient with epilepsy. Neurology 1998;51(4):1224–5. Available at: http://www.ncbi.nlm.nih.gov/pubmed/9781571.

76. Iriarte J, Artieda J, Alegre M, et al. Spasm of the sternocleidomastoid muscle induced by vagal nerve stimulation. Neurology 2001;57(12):2319–20. Available at: http://www.ncbi.nlm.nih.gov/pubmed/11756622.

77. Kim W, Clancy RR, Liu GT. Horner syndrome associated with implantation of a vagus nerve stimulator. Am J Ophthalmol 2001;131(3):383–4. Available at: http://www.ncbi.nlm.nih.gov/pubmed/11239877.

78. Ramsay RE, Uthman BM, Augustinsson LE, et al. Vagus nerve stimulation for treatment of partial seizures: 2. Safety, side effects, and tolerability. First International Vagus Nerve Stimulation Study Group. Epilepsia 1994;35(3):627–36. Available at: http://www.ncbi.nlm.nih.gov/pubmed/8026409.

79. Smyth MD, Tubbs RS, Bebin EM, et al. Complications of chronic vagus nerve stimulation for epilepsy in children. J Neurosurg 2003;99(3):500–3.

80. Labiner DM, Ahern GL. Vagus nerve stimulation therapy in depression and epilepsy: therapeutic parameter settings. Acta Neurol Scand 2007;115(1):23–33.

81. Denski KM, Labiner DM. Should I offer vagus nerve stimulation as part of my neurology practice? Neurol Clin Pract 2014;4(4):313–8.

82. Lundy DS, Casiano RR, Landy HJ, et al. Effects of vagal nerve stimulation on laryngeal function. J Voice 1993;7(4):359–64.

83. Koutroumanidis M, Hennessy MJ, Binnie CD, et al. Aggravation of partial epilepsy and emergence of new seizure type during treatment with VNS. Neurology 2000; 55(6):892–3. Available at: http://www.ncbi.nlm.nih.gov/pubmed/10994021.

84. Arhan E, Serdaroğlu A, Hirfanoğlu T, et al. Aggravation of seizures and status epilepticus after vagal nerve stimulation therapy: the first pediatric case and review of the literature. Childs Nerv Syst 2018;34(9):1799–801.

85. Tatum WO, Helmers SL. Vagus nerve stimulation and magnet use: optimizing benefits. Epilepsy Behav 2009;15(3):299–302.

86. de Jonge JC, Melis GI, Gebbink TA, et al. Safety of a dedicated brain MRI protocol in patients with a vagus nerve stimulator. Epilepsia 2014;55(11):e112–5.

87. Cyberonics. MRI Guidelines for VNS Therapy [PDF file]. Cardion Website. 2014. Available at: http://www.cardion.cz/data/mri-kompatibilita/vns-terapie.pdf. Accessed March 25, 2019.

88. Cyberonics. MRI safety. LivaNova Website. 2019. Available at: https://us. livanova.cyberonics.com/learn-more/mri-safety. Accessed March 25, 2019.

89. Cyberonics. MRI scan Conditions (group B). LivaNova Website. 2017. Available at: https://us.livanova.cyberonics.com/healthcare-professionals/mri/question-2/ answer-b. Accessed March 25, 2019.

Recurrent Laryngeal Nerve Stimulator

Andreas H. Mueller, MD[a],*, Claus Pototschnig, MD[b]

KEYWORDS

- Larynx • Vocal fold paralysis/paresis therapy • Implantable neurostimulator
- Neurostimulation • Laryngeal pacing

KEY POINTS

- Dynamic therapy options for remobilization of at least 1 side in bilateral vocal fold paralysis could overcome the deficits of the surgical procedures currently used.
- Electromyographic detection of residual innervation or pathologic, ideally synkinetic laryngeal reinnervation is the most important prerequisite for concepts of recurrent laryngeal nerve stimulators.
- Preclinical and initial clinical studies have proven the safety and efficacy of laryngeal neurostimulation. Patients can currently only be implanted with laryngeal pacemakers (LP) within the framework of clinical studies until the LP systems are approved by the responsible authorities.
- Because of its minimally invasive character, LP systems can be used also in patients with comorbidities and those who reject more invasive surgery.
- Currently, the synchronization of LP systems with respiration is a research focus.

INTRODUCTION

Most commonly, recurrent laryngeal nerve paralysis (RLNP) has an idiopathic or iatrogenic origin. The most frequent iatrogenic causes include thyroid or cervical spine surgery.[1] Occasionally, RLNP is due to tumors, strokes, or neural inflammations. When the recurrent laryngeal nerve (RLN) damage is limited (eg, neurapraxia or axonotmesis), the vocal fold (VF) mobility can recover within 6 to 12 months after RLN injury.[2] On the contrary, severe nerve lesions (eg, neurotmesis) may result in a progressive VF muscle atrophy or lead to impaired (paresis) to completely inhibited (paralysis)

Disclosure Statement: The authors received travel grants from MED-EL Elektromedizinische Geraete GmbH, Innsbruck, Austria to present clinical trial results on laryngeal pacing at scientific conferences. MED-EL financially supported part of the research performed by SRH Wald-Klinikum on laryngeal pacing.
The authors received no honorarium by MED-EL. They have no other financial relationships, or conflicts of interest to disclose.
[a] Otorhinolaryngology, SRH Wald-Klinikum, Strasse des Friedens 122, Gera 07548, Germany;
[b] Otorhinolaryngology, Innsbruck University Hospital, Anichstrasse 35, Innsbruck 6020, Austria
* Corresponding author.
E-mail address: andreas.mueller@srh.de

Otolaryngol Clin N Am 53 (2020) 145–156
https://doi.org/10.1016/j.otc.2019.09.009
0030-6665/20/© 2019 Elsevier Inc. All rights reserved.

VF mobility. Persistent VF paresis and paralysis (VFP) without atrophy are generally accompanied by a relevant degree of dysfunctional (eg, misdirected) reinnervation of the laryngeal muscles that, although preserving a certain extent of muscular bulk and VF tonus, yet impedes the restoration of normal volitional VF activity.[3]

Although unilateral VFP (UVFP) mainly affects the voice quality, bilateral VFP (BVFP) is frequently associated with the development of potentially life-threatening dyspnea.

UVFP is most commonly conservatively treated by voice therapy. VF augmentation, arytenoid adduction, and laryngeal framework surgery are limited to more severe cases for which voice therapy is unable to reach satisfactory results for the patient. However, patients requiring a complete restoration of their voice quality, such as singers and professional speakers, may be less satisfied with treatments that compromise vocal pitch or the synchronicity of the mucosal wave movements. Particularly for such patients, neuromuscular rehabilitation, like nonselective reinnervation[4,5] and, in the future, neurostimulation,[6] may become the most beneficial and satisfactory UVFP treatments.

BVFP occurrence is far less frequent than UVFP (<1–1.7 cases per 100,000).[7] Most commonly, BVFP is surgically treated. Endolaryngeal glottal enlargement is considered the golden-standard therapy for this condition, whereas tracheostomy is usually limited to emergency cases. In both cases, the surgical restoration of the air patency is achieved to the expense of the voice quality.[8]

There is therefore a great need for new treatments that improve breathing without worsening the voice. Research in neuromuscular therapies for at least partial restoration of the VF mobility, and in selective laryngeal reinnervation by grafting phrenic nerve and Ansa cervicalis branches,[9] has been fostered since the late 1970s.[10]

The aim of this article is to provide an accurate overview on the recent progressing of the research in neurostimulators for RLNP (laryngeal pacing) and offer a realist outlook on its clinical prospective.

SURFACE STIMULATION

Transcutaneous electrical muscle *stimulation (TES)* is particularly effective in stimulating superficial muscles closest to the skin surface. For instance, TES of the submental or prelaryngeal cervical region by means of adhesive surface electrodes has been successfully tried for dysphagia treatment. Unfortunately, because the internal laryngeal muscles are located deep in the neck and electrically isolated by the laryngeal framework, TES was proven not very successful in restoring VF mobility following RLN injury in the past.[11]

TES effectiveness is predicted to be linked to the pulse frequency and duration of the applied electrical stimulus. Although frequencies greater than 100 kHz are used to heat the tissue in physical therapy, they do not associate with effective muscle contractions. On the contrary, TES with sufficient current intensity at low frequencies (ie, up to 1 kHz) has been shown to elicit an effective muscle contraction. Seifpanahi and colleagues[12] showed that short-term impulses (100-Hz pulse rate with biphasic pulse duration of 200 millisecond) elicit VF movements in healthy volunteers. Schneider-Stickler and colleagues[13] recently published a preliminary work showing similar results in UVFP patients.

Long before attempting to induce VF movements, TES was used to reduce VF atrophy after RLN injury.[14] Because denervated muscles are less sensitive to electrical stimulation than healthy muscle fibers, higher currents and longer pulse durations are required to adequately elicit their response.[15] However, the current intensity necessary to elicit such response may also cause skin irritations, pain, and an undesired current spread toward the overlaying strap muscles. In conclusion, a critical and accurate clinical evaluation is necessary to demonstrate the clinical effectiveness of TES in RLNP.

After the reinnervation process following RLNP, muscles can be effectively stimulated by *neuromuscular electrical stimulation (NMES)* targeting their innervating fibers. Because nerve fibers have a significantly lower excitatory threshold than muscles, effective NMES can be achieved with a current intensity 10 to 100 times lower than that required for muscle stimulation. Because of the dense innervating system of the neck muscle, NMES performed by means of a bipolar needle with localized current spread is expected to successfully induce a very selective laryngeal stimulation. However, because needle stimulation is preferentially used in diagnostics and never for therapy, NMES-based treatments are usually applied, similarly to TES, by means of adhesive surface electrodes. If the patient is asked to perform voluntary activities during the NMES administration, the targeted muscles seem to show an increase in their tonus. The successful use of NMES in UVFP patients was described by Ptok and Strack.[16] The investigators showed that in a prospective randomized study, voice therapy combined with NMES was more effective than voice therapy alone in restoring the patient's voice quality. In addition, Garcia Perez and colleagues[17] showed in another prospective clinical study that NMES application during sustained phonation accelerated the recovery from UVFP symptoms.

There is sparse evidence of patients claiming a lasting therapeutic effect of the NMES long after the stimulation. However, the substantial lack of knowledge about the influence of peripheral nerve stimulation on neuronal plasticity underlying the ability to regain some degree of VF functionality has so far prevented a scientifically sound demonstration of such NMES effect.

HISTORY OF LARYNGEAL NEUROSTIMULATION WITH IMPLANTED ELECTRODES

The first experiments concerning laryngeal neurostimulation were described by Zealear and Dedo[18] in an article published in 1977. The acute experiment was conducted on dogs with artificially denervated laryngeal muscles. After unilateral dissection of the superior laryngeal nerve (SLN), the affected cricothyroid muscle (CT) was electrically stimulated synchronously with the physiologic movements of the contralateral CT innervated by an intact SLN. Shortly thereafter, Bergmann's group was the first to implant electrodes into an artificially paralyzed posterior cricoarytenoid muscle (PCA) in a dog model. The stimulation-elicited VF abduction was synchronized with respiration for the first time in 1984 by means of an external chest strap sensor (closed loop).[19] The stimulation system was the *first chronically implanted laryngeal pacemaker* and was found to be stable in 4 of 6 dogs for a follow-up period between 3 and 11 months. In 2 of 6 cases, the cables broke within 3 months after implantation because of the significant mechanical stress of the implanted region (ie, the neck).[20] The work of Obert and colleagues[21] showed that, at least in dogs, it is possible to completely restore VF abduction in bilaterally denervated PCAs by single-sided implantation of a bipolar single-stranded electrode. Using the same model, Otto and colleagues[22] showed that the diaphragm electromyographic (EMG) signal can be used as a respiratory trigger for PCA stimulation. Zrunek and colleagues[23] showed in a sheep model that long-term low-frequency direct electrical stimulation of chronically denervated PCAs causes a change of the muscle fibers from type 2 (fast) to type 1 (slow). Kano and Sasaki[24] thoroughly investigated the influence of the electrode material and the stimulation parameters on the reduction of electrical charge accumulation at the electrode tip and the associated corrosion risks in a canine model, using a pair of platinum-tungsten coil electrodes. In short, they inserted the electrode pair into the PCA at a distance of 2 mm from each other and delivered biphasic pulses of 2 milliseconds to elicit VF abduction. Sanders[15] systematically investigated the belly structure of the canine PCA, the abduction effect of various stimulation parameters, and the effects of the electrode insertion site and orientation to the PCA fibers have on the stimulation. He also investigated histopathologic changes after long-term stimulation.

In 1989, Bergmann received the authorization by the responsible ethics commission in East Germany for the first-in-human clinical trial to evaluate the efficacy of laryngeal pacing in humans. However, because of safety and performance concerns, he decided to abort the study without enrolling any patients. Shortly thereafter, Germany was reunited, and fundamental changes in the health care system led to the discontinuation of the study.[25] Later, the first-in-human multicentric study was conducted in the United States in 1995 by Zealear in collaboration with an international team. This study selected patients suffering from BVFP, but without life-threatening respiratory issues, because they have all been tracheotomized before their enrollment in the study. A standard pain-therapy implant (Itrel II; Medtronic, Minneapolis, MN, USA) with 3- or 4-channel spinal cord electrodes was used as an implantable pulse generator.[26] This proof-of-principle study was a milestone in the history of laryngeal pacing and provided initial evidence of the safety and efficacy of this treatment option. However, because the study also exposed significant problems with the chosen nondedicated laryngeal neurostimulator, such as electrode corrosion and off-target stimulation, clinical research with such a device was discontinued.

RECENT RECURRENT LARYNGEAL NERVE STIMULATOR CONCEPTS

An accurate literature review of clinical trials aiming to evaluate the potential benefits of surface electrical stimulation for BVFP patients and of preclinical trials in animal models with the aim of determining the optimal configuration of implantable neuromuscular stimulators clearly show that direct electrical muscle stimulation should be avoided in favor of neuromuscular stimulation. The lower current intensities of NMES also derisk electrode corrosion, an event repeatedly observed and reported in Zealear's works, and avoid the occurrence of adverse events, such as inflammation and burns of the tissue targeted by stimulation. Another direct consequence of the NMES principle is that it is not applicable to completely denervated laryngeal muscles that would respond only to stimulations with higher current intensities. Accordingly, neurostimulation therapies for BVFP should be exclusively considered for patients showing a partial, misdirected, or dysfunctional reinnervation of at least 1 PCA, even if unable to support the restoration of the volitional mobility of the respective VF. Granted that the stimulation is applied on the terminal branches innervating the target muscle rather than on the trunk of the RLN, even aberrant reinnervation is sufficient to ensure the efficacy of this treatment. Nonroutine options, like immediate RLN reconstruction in iatrogenic dissection[27] or nonselective reinnervation of the internal laryngeal muscles with the ansa cervicalis[6] in cases of progressive muscle atrophy, can improve the innervation status. Patients treated either way may become future candidates for the implantation of laryngeal pacemakers.

The PCA innervation pattern has a strong individual component that determines the position and concentration of the distal RLN fibers, responsible for the VF abduction. The points on the PCA with a high concentration of such fibers are known as "hotspots"[28] and are generally located in the lower lateral quadrant of the muscle. This is the preferred target for test stimulation, a technique used to identify the PCA hotspot that, if electrical stimulated, elicits an effective VF abduction. Targeting a specific

PCA hot-spot (**Fig. 1**) rather than applying the stimulation on a larger portion of the PCA by means of grid electrodes should be preferred because of (a) the less invasive electrode placement procedure,[29] which would eliminate the need of open-laryngeal surgery, (b) the low current intensity, and (c) the minimized risk of injuring surrounding laryngeal tissues during electrode implantation, which prevents the formation of scars that would severely impair an effective VF abduction stimulation. A major challenge for electrical stimulation conducted on the PCA hot-spot is the long-lasting anchoring of the electrode, which is subject to continuous and prolonged mechanical stress owing to head and neck movements. Previous preclinical trials conducted in minipigs confirmed that the technique used for the placement and the anchoring of the electrode should be carefully chosen in order to avoid later displacements or breakages.[30] The use of appropriate and dedicated tools for the electrode implantation further improves the electrode stability over time.

In order to avoid the occurrence of corrosion problems as those described by Zealear and colleagues,[26] the electrode tip placed into the PCA hot-spot should be designed taking in account the potential effects of current distribution, electrical charge density, and chemical resistance.

An optimal laryngeal pacemaker should support biphasic stimulation with a range of the most effective amplitudes, pulse widths, and frequencies for pathologically reinnervated PCAs. In addition, it should allow individual-specific fitting of the stimulation parameters to accommodate the real needs of each patient.

It is expected that if the stimulation can be synchronized with the patient's respiratory cycle, the effectiveness of the laryngeal pacemaker will further increase. In order to develop a new generation of such perfected laryngeal pacemakers, it is of paramount

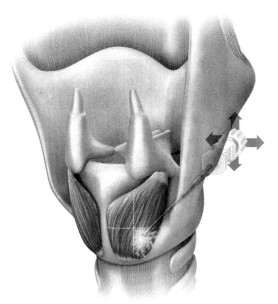

Fig. 1. Search for the "Hot-Spot" in the PCA muscle with the insertion tool of the LP System (*red arrows*) = change of direction of the tool; Hot-spot (*green flashes*) = a point in the PCA whose electrical stimulation leads to a laryngoscopically verifiable and reproducible vocal fold abduction, which is usually located in the lower lateral quadrant (*dotted quadrant division*) (MED-EL, Innsbruck, Austria).

importance to find a precise and accurate sensor, capable of adapting the stimulation to the respiratory effort of the patient. The external chest wall sensor used for polysomnography or an implantable sensor such as those used in combination with hypoglossal nerve stimulators theoretically meet such requirements. However, although their performance is high in lying and almost motionless patients, it severely decreases in actively moving subjects. The authors' team is currently investigating the performance of sensors based on the use of the inspiratory EMG signal of the parasternal musculature as the most suitable alternative to such a sensor. De Troyer and Sampson[31] described for the first time in 1982 the correlation between the activity of the intercostal muscles directly adjacent to the sternum, also known as parasternal muscles, and inspiration. They showed that increased activity of the parasternal EMG was elicited by both thoracic and relaxed diaphragmatic respiration. The parasternal EMG signal has a rostrocaudal gradient from the first to the fifth intercostal interspace. The parasternal EMG signal of the first to third interspace, for instance, is recordable only within the first 10% of the inspiratory cycle.[32] In a preliminary study (Claus Pototschnig, Christian Denk, 2017, unpublished data) conducted at the University Hospital Innsbruck on 9 healthy volunteers, the authors' group investigated the potentiality of a sensor based on the EMG signal recorded on the second and third intercostal space by means of hooked-wire percutaneous electrodes placed under sonographic guidance (**Fig. 2**). The precision and accuracy of the EMG signal was evaluated with the patient performing different movements, such moving the arms or heavily breathing while standing, walking, sitting, and speaking. The results showed that movements of the upper half of the body severely interfered with the EMG signal. Further hindering effects were found to be a body mass index greater than 35 and upper chest muscle tension. Although in unmoving, standing patients the EMG could be reproducibly detected, this was impossible in patients actively moving the upper half of their body. This was due to the presence of motion-linked artifacts in the signal as well as to the acute setting of the study. Further clinical trials in a more stable setting and in larger cohorts are currently in progress in order to better evaluate the value of parasternal EMG as a potential respiratory sensor for improved generations of laryngeal pacemakers.

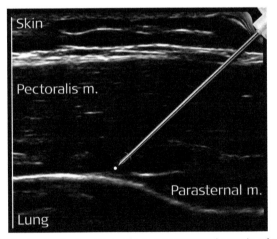

Fig. 2. Placement of a hooked-wire electrode in a parasternal muscle of a volunteer under ultrasound guidance to investigate the synchronicity of activation of this muscle with inspiration and the influence of movement artifacts; see the neighborhood of the target (*white dot*) to the lung, the pectoralis muscle overlays the parasternal muscle, its contraction may affect the EMG signal (MED-EL, Innsbruck, Austria).

SELECTION OF MOST SUITABLE CANDIDATES FOR LARYNGEAL NERVE STIMULATORS

Because of its characteristics, laryngeal pacing will not be effective for all the BVFP patients. Thus, a careful selection of the most suitable recipients is necessary to exploit the benefits of such a therapy. In particular, the optimal candidates will meet the following conditions[33]:

1. Suffering from permanent BVFP correlating with moderate to severe respiratory problems during physical exertion that are not linked to the presence of comorbidities
2. The PCAs undergoing electrode implantation show a muscle bulk sufficient to guarantee a functional response of the respective VF (abduction) to the stimulation
3. The cricoarytenoid joints are intact and mobile
4. At least the PCAs are partially (synkinetically) reinnervated.

The compliance with condition 1 should be verified by medical history review, respiratory test (eg, spirometry), and videolaryngoscopy; the latter, supplemented, if necessary, with a panendoscopy, should also be used to verify compliance with condition 3. Compliance with condition 2 and 4 should be verified by means of test stimulation with or without Laryngeal EMG (LEMG) and videolaryngoscopy.

In addition to compliance with the aforementioned criteria, the candidates should be willing to accept the risks linked to surgical device implantation, such as the possibility that the electrode should be explanted for breakages or lack of functionality. Depending on the characteristics of the implanted laryngeal nerve stimulator, the patient should be informed about the MRI compatibility of the device.

Although, depending on the patient's VF conditions and the presence of previous VF surgeries, the laryngeal pacemaker electrode can be implanted unilaterally or bilaterally, it is expected that the bilateral will deliver better results than unilateral implantation in terms of both respiratory improvement and voice preservation. Also, patients initially unilaterally implanted can receive a second electrode on the contralateral VF at a later point, if compliant with the selection criteria.

Based on evidence from scientific literature and the authors' personal experience, they do not expect that the duration of the BVFP would negatively affect the laryngeal pacemaker performance as long as all the selection criteria listed above are met. However, laryngeal pacemaker implantation should be considered 6 to 12 months after the onset of the BVFP, in order to confirm that such condition is permanent and likely not subject to natural recovery. The idea of an early implantation immediately after BVFP onset, as previously advocated by Zealear and colleagues [34] and Al-Majed and colleagues,[35] of supporting the selective and correct reinnervation of the adductor and adductor muscle in the early stages of reinnervation is unfortunately not backed by sufficiently sound evidence.

PRELIMINARY CLINICAL RESULTS WITH LARYNGEAL PACING: SAFETY AND PERFORMANCE OF MED-EL LARYNGEAL PACEMAKERS SYSTEM

The authors' team has been actively contributing to the design and development of a dedicated laryngeal pacing system, known by its project title "Laryngeal Pacemaker (LP) System," for the treatment of BVFP patients. The LP System is a medical device currently under preclinical investigations, manufactured by the Austrian company, MED-EL Elektromedizinische Geraete, headquartered in Innsbruck, based on the concept elaborated by this company, and the ENT departments of SRH Wald Klinikum Gera, and the University Hospitals of Innsbruck and Würzburg.[29,30] The LP System has been conceived to require minimally invasive surgery for its implantation (**Fig. 3**). The electrode design has been devised to prevent irreversible laryngeal tissue damage, even in the case of explantation. The LP System is an example of reversible treatment, differently from glottal enlargement, that causes a permanent change in the laryngeal structure. In case of lack of benefits, the patient may decide to permanently switch off or remove the implant and undergo another surgical or conservative therapy that will not be affected at all by the earlier LP System implantation.

The LP System was investigated for the first time in humans in a clinical trial conducted between 2012 and 2014 by the 3 hospitals involved in its design and development. The study was approved by the relevant ethics committees and national competent authorities and enrolled 9 patients. The postimplantation follow-up period of the study was 6 months. The study investigated the safety of the LP System and of the implantation procedure as well as the performance of the device in terms of respiratory function, voice quality, physical activity support, and quality of life.[36] All patients were exclusively unilaterally implanted. In 1 case, it was impossible to fix the electrode in a sufficiently stable way, and thus, it was early explanted, and the patient was consequently withdrawn from the study. Another patient was withdrawn after becoming pregnant and passively followed up for the entire study period. Seven of 9 subjects completed the entire follow-up period. The implanted patients showed excellent compliance with the study requirement and the LP System handling (**Fig. 4**). The 2 patients with an open tracheostoma before implantation were decannulated within the follow-up period. Upon postimplantation activation, all the patients showed increased values of normalized peak expiratory and inspiratory flow, comparable with those observed with glottal enlargement, but without the accompanying voice quality impairment typical for this latter treatment. No swallow problems were observed for the entire follow-up period.

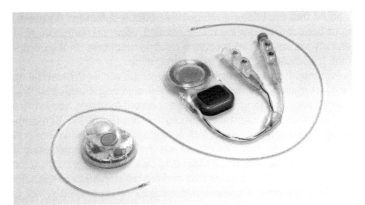

Fig. 3. Laryngeal Pacemaker System (LP System). The *LP Processor* (left in the figure) consists of a control unit powered by a battery, and the coil for the inductive transmission of signals and energy to the LP implant. The LP Processor has a single control button to adapt the characteristics of the stimulation burst frequency to meet the specific needs of the users and their different situations. The *LP Implant* (right in the figure) consists of a titanium housing that protects the internal electronics, an inductive coil to receive signals from the external LP Processor, and two connectors. The 3 French soft *LP Electrode* (s-shaped in the figure) is a bipolar, linear electrode with a length of 30 cm. The lead of the LP Electrode consists of a spiral arrangement of the wires in a silicon lead body. The ring and tip electrodes are used to deliver the stimulation on the nerve branches of the posterior cricoarytenoid (PCA) muscle, whereas the active helical electrode tip is used to fix and anchor the LP Electrode onto the PCA muscle (MED-EL, Innsbruck, Austria).

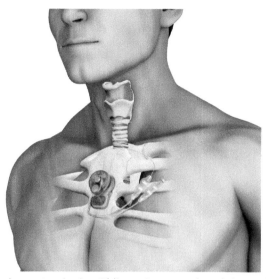

Fig. 4. Laryngeal Pacing system in situ. Oblique view to neck and chest with one of the two possible *LP Electrodes* inserted into the left sided PCA muscle; the green illuminated sections of the electrode symbolize the stimulation impulses sent to the larynx; The *LP Implant* is placed in a subcutaneous pocket onto the sternum and coupled to the one LP Electrode on the lateral chest wall via one of the two *LP Implant connectors*; The *LP Processor* is kept on the skin over the LP Implant by magnetic attraction (MED-EL, Innsbruck, Austria).

Both Short Form-36 and Glasgow Benefit Inventory showed improved results compared with the baseline, at least concerning the mental component of the questionnaires.

Although very promising, these results are merely exploratory, and the authors are planning larger cohort studies to confirm these preliminary outcomes.

The most striking result of the LP System was the complete preservation of the voice. In a world based on communication, the loss of voice quality has a severe impact on both the private and the professional life of the BVFP patients.[37,38] Thus, the LP System can become a very attractive alternative to glottal enlargement. In the authors' first study, they showed that although before implantation, all the enrolled patents suffered from moderate voice quality impairment according to the results of the Voice Handicap Index-12, the LP System implantation did not further negatively affect their voice. On the contrary, over time they saw a nonsignificant trend toward voice quality improvement that should be confirmed in larger cohort studies.

The LP System evaluated in the authors' first study was not synchronized to the patients' respiratory cycle. However, it never interfered with either phonation or swallowing, suggesting that the remaining VF adduction of a synkinetically reinnervated larynx is still able to effectively override the PCA stimulation during activities requiring the glottal gap closure.

SUMMARY

Electrical stimulation of the RLN is a promising therapeutic approach with the potentiality to overcome the shortcomings of conventional surgical glottal enlargement. Although synkinetic or aberrant reinnervation is commonly considered an unfavorable condition, its presence is valuable to ensure the clinical applicability of laryngeal pacemakers. Thus, the effective selection of patients who can really profit from LP implantation demands the implementation of new diagnostic tools based on tests capable of reliably detecting the presence of residual reinnervation on at least 1 VF. Preclinical animal trials and premarket clinical studies confirmed the safety of laryngeal pacing and provided preliminary evidence of its clinical performance. Currently, a major research focus in the development of improved LPs is the synchronization of the stimulation with the patient's respiration cycle.

REFERENCES

1. Reiter R, Hoffmann TK, Rotter N, et al. Etiology, diagnosis, differential diagnosis and therapy of vocal fold paralysis. Laryngorhinootologie 2014;93(3):161–73 [in German].
2. Husain S, Sadoughi B, Mor N, et al. Time course of recovery of iatrogenic vocal fold paralysis. Laryngoscope 2019;129(5):1159–63.
3. Rubin AD, Sataloff RT. Vocal fold paresis and paralysis. Otolaryngol Clin North Am 2007;40(5):1109–31, viii–ix.
4. Wang W, Chen D, Chen S, et al. Laryngeal reinnervation using ansa cervicalis for thyroid surgery-related unilateral vocal fold paralysis: a long-term outcome analysis of 237 cases. PLoS One 2011;6(4):e19128.
5. Crumley RL, Izdebski K. Voice quality following laryngeal reinnervation by ansa hypoglossi transfer. Laryngoscope 1986;96(6):611–6.
6. Mueller AH, Klinge K. RLN paralysis–update on reinnervation and neurostimulation. Arch Med Res 2018;6(5):1–12.
7. Nawka T, Gugatschka M, Kolmel JC, et al. Therapy of bilateral vocal fold paralysis: real world data of an international multi-center registry. PLoS One 2019;14(4):e0216096.
8. Benninger MS, Xiao R, Osborne K, et al. Outcomes following cordotomy by co-blation for bilateral vocal fold immobility. JAMA Otolaryngol Head Neck Surg 2018;144(2):149–55.
9. Marina MB, Marie JP, Birchall MA. Laryngeal reinnervation for bilateral vocal fold paralysis. Curr Opin Otolaryngol Head Neck Surg 2011;19(6):434–8.
10. Zealear DL, Dedo HH. Control of paralyzed axial muscles by electrical stimulation. Trans Sect Ophthalmol Am Acad Ophthalmol Otolaryngol 1977;84(2):310.
11. Humbert I, Poletto C, Saxon KG, et al. The effect of surface electrical stimulation on vocal fold position. Laryngoscope 2008;118:14–9.
12. Seifpanahi S, Izadi F, Jamshidi AA, et al. Effects of transcutaneous electrical stimulation on vocal folds adduction. Eur Arch Otorhinolaryngol 2017;274(9):3423–8.
13. Schneider-Stickler B, Leonhard M, Krenn M et al. Selective surface stimulation of unilateral vocal fold paralysis. Laryngo-Rhino-Otologie 2018;97(S02): 17 - 17. https://doi.org/10.1055/s-0038-163977309.–12. Mai 2018, Musik- und Kongresshalle (MuK) Lübeck, Germany.
14. Iakovleva I, Iliutovich GM, Iuvalova ND. On the use of sinusoidal low-frequency modulated currents in vocal disorders in patients with paralysis and paresis of the laryngeal muscles. Vestn Otorinolaringol 1965;27(5):93–8 [in Russian].
15. Sanders I. Electrical stimulation of laryngeal muscle. Otolaryngol Clin North Am 1991;24(5):1253–74.
16. Ptok M, Strack D. Electrical stimulation-supported voice exercises are superior to voice exercise therapy alone in patients with unilateral recurrent laryngeal nerve paresis: results from a prospective, randomized clinical trial. Muscle Nerve 2008;38(2):1005–11.

17. Garcia Perez A, Hernandez Lopez X, Valadez Jimenez VM, et al. Synchronous electrical stimulation of laryngeal muscles: an alternative for enhancing recovery of unilateral recurrent laryngeal nerve paralysis. J Voice 2014;28(4):524.e1-7.

18. Zealear DL, Dedo HH. Control of paralysed axial muscles by electrical stimulation. Acta Otolaryngol 1977;83(5–6):514–27.

19. Bergmann K, Warzel H, Eckhardt HU, et al. Respiratory rhythmically regulated electrical stimulation of paralyzed laryngeal muscles. Laryngoscope 1984; 94(10):1376–80.

20. Bergmann K, Warzel H, Eckhardt HU, et al. Long-term implantation of a system of electrical stimulation of paralyzed laryngeal muscles in dogs. Laryngoscope 1988;98(4):455–9.

21. Obert PM, Young KA, Tobey DN. Use of direct posterior cricoarytenoid stimulation in laryngeal paralysis. Arch Otolaryngol 1984;110(2):88–92.

22. Otto RA, Templer J, Davis W, et al. Coordinated electrical pacing of vocal cord abductors in recurrent laryngeal nerve paralysis. Otolaryngol Head Neck Surg 1985;93(5):634–8.

23. Zrunek M, Carraro U, Catani C, et al. Functional electrostimulation of the denervated posticus muscle in an animal experiment: histo- and biochemical results. Laryngol Rhinol Otol (Stuttg) 1986;65(11):621–7 [in German].

24. Kano S, Sasaki CT. Pacing parameters of the canine posterior cricoarytenoid muscle. Ann Otol Rhinol Laryngol 1991;100(7):584–8.

25. Bergmann K. History of the Laryngeal Pacing in the GDR in the 80th. In. 2nd Neurolaryngology Workshop for Experts ed. Jena/Gera: FSU Jena; 2015.

26. Zealear DL, Billante CR, Courey MS, et al. Reanimation of the paralyzed human larynx with an implantable electrical stimulation device. Laryngoscope 2003; 113(7):1149–56.

27. Zabrodsky M, Boucek J, Kastner J, et al. Immediate revision in patients with bilateral recurrent laryngeal nerve palsy after thyroid and parathyroid surgery. How worthy is it? Acta Otorhinolaryngol Ital 2012;32(4):222–8.

28. Zealear DL, Rainey CL, Jerles ML, et al. Technical approach for reanimation of the chronically denervated larynx by means of functional electrical stimulation. Ann Otol Rhinol Laryngol 1994;103(9):705–12.

29. Forster G, Arnold D, Bischoff SJ, et al. Laryngeal pacing in minipigs: in vivo test of a new minimal invasive transcricoidal electrode insertion method for functional electrical stimulation of the PCA. Eur Arch Otorhinolaryngol 2013;270(1):225–31.

30. Foerster G, Arnold D, Bischoff S, et al. Pre-clinical evaluation of a minimally invasive laryngeal pacemaker system in mini-pig. Eur Arch Otorhinolaryngol 2016; 273(1):151–8.

31. De Troyer A, Sampson MG. Activation of the parasternal intercostals during breathing efforts in human subjects. J Appl Physiol Respir Environ Exerc Physiol 1982;52(3):524–9.

32. Gandevia SC, Hudson AL, Gorman RB, et al. Spatial distribution of inspiratory drive to the parasternal intercostal muscles in humans. J Physiol 2006;573(Pt 1):263–75.

33. Mueller AH, Foerster G. Who are suitable candidates for laryngeal pacing? Paper presented at: 7th Congress of the European Laryngological Society. Barcelona, Spain, May 29–31, 2008.

34. Zealear DL, Mainthia R, Li Y, et al. Stimulation of denervated muscle promotes selective reinnervation, prevents synkinesis, and restores function. Laryngoscope 2014;124(5):E180–7.

35. Al-Majed AA, Neumann CM, Brushart TM, et al. Brief electrical stimulation pro-motes the speed and accuracy of motor axonal regeneration. J Neurosci 2000; 20(7):2602–8.
36. Mueller AH, Hagen R, Foerster G, et al. Laryngeal pacing via an implantable stim-ulator for the rehabilitation of subjects suffering from bilateral vocal fold paralysis: a prospective first-in-human study. Laryngoscope 2016;126(8):1810–6.
37. Mueller AH, Hagen R, Pototschnig C, et al. Laryngeal pacing for bilateral vocal fold paralysis: voice and respiratory aspects. Laryngoscope 2017;127(8): 1838–44.
38. Nawka T, Sittel C, Arens C, et al. Voice and respiratory outcomes after permanent transoral surgery of bilateral vocal fold paralysis. Laryngoscope 2015;125(12): 2749–55.

Hypoglossal Nerve (Cranial Nerve XII) Stimulation

Jason L. Yu, MD[a], Erica R. Thaler, MD[b],*

KEYWORDS

- Upper airway stimulation • Hypoglossal nerve stimulation • Obstructive sleep apnea

KEY POINTS

- The anatomy and physiology of the hypoglossal nerve allow for easy surgical access and tolerable neurostimulation.
- Hypoglossal nerve stimulation is currently the only upper airway stimulation (UAS) device approved for the treatment of obstructive sleep apnea (OSA).
- UAS has shown a treatment success rate of with improvements in OSA severity, sleepiness, and sleep quality of life, with 94% of patients ultimately being satisfied with surgery and therapy.
- Future studies will look at the effects of UAS on medical outcomes in the treatment of OSA as well as in improving the understanding of the pathophysiology of OSA to better select patients for surgery.

INTRODUCTION

The hypoglossal nerve, also known as cranial nerve XII, innervates the intrinsic muscles of the tongue as well as 3 extrinsic tongue muscles: the genioglossus, the styloglossus, and the hyoglossus. The fourth extrinsic muscle of the tongue, the palatoglossus, has separate innervation by cranial nerve X. The hypoglossal nerve originates from the hypoglossal nucleus within the medulla oblongata of the brainstem. It courses along the posterior fossa of the skull and exits the skull base through its own foramen, the hypoglossal canal, and enters the neck. It descends into the neck deep between the internal carotid artery and the internal jugular vein deep to the posterior belly of the digastric muscle. It crosses over the occipital artery branch of the external carotid artery and progresses anteriorly in the deep lateral neck inferior medial to the digastric tendon. There it turns superiorly, running deep to the mylohyoid muscles. Once deep to the mylohyoid muscle, the nerve branches into lateral and

[a] Division of Sleep Medicine, Hospital of the University of Pennsylvania, 3624 Market Street Suite 201, Philadelphia, PA 19104, USA; [b] Department of Otorhinolaryngology, Hospital of the University of Pennsylvania, 3400 Spruce St. 5th floor Silverstein Bldg, Philadelphia, PA 19104, USA
* Corresponding author.
E-mail address: Erica.thaler@uphs.upenn.edu

Otolaryngol Clin N Am 53 (2020) 157–169
https://doi.org/10.1016/j.otc.2019.09.010
0030-6665/20/© 2019 Elsevier Inc. All rights reserved.

medical branches to innervate its target musculature (**Fig. 1**). The lateral branches innervate the styloglossus and hyoglossus muscles, while the medial branch innervates the genioglossus and the intrinsic tongue musculature (transverse and vertical muscles).[1,2]

The tongue consists of intrinsic and extrinsic musculature, which is innervated primarily by the hypoglossal nerve save the palatoglossus, which is innervated by the vagus nerve. The extrinsic muscles: the hyoglossus, genioglossus, palatoglossus, and styloglossus, have insertions onto bone and function to protrude (genioglossus) or retract (styloglossus, hyoglossus, palatoglossus) the tongue. The intrinsic muscles: the transverse, vertical, and longitudinal, do not insert onto bone but rather originate and insert within the tongue itself and function to stiffen or shape the tongue.[3]

There are numerous factors that make the hypoglossal nerve an ideal target for surgical stimulation. Its course makes it easily accessible to surgeons without major risk to other structures in the head and neck, including other cranial nerves and major blood vessels. At its distal portion, the nerve branches allow for selective innervation of different target musculature. The nerve is also a general somatic efferent nerve with sole motor function, and thus, activation will not lead to sensory input causing pain.

Hypoglossal nerve stimulation (HGNS) is currently the only neurostimulation device approved for the treatment of obstructive sleep apnea (OSA).[4] OSA is estimated to affect up to 22 million Americans and is associated with significant health morbidity and mortality.[5] OSA is caused by the narrowing and/or collapse of the upper airway in breathing during sleep, leading to hypoxia during sleep as well as arousals from sleep. Periods of complete obstruction are called apneas, whereas periods of airway narrowing significant enough to cause desaturation or arousal are called hypopneas. The apnea-hypopnea index (AHI) is a calculation of how many of these events occur per hour over the course of the night. An AHI greater than 5 events per hour is considered diagnostic for OSA.[6]

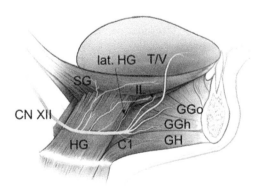

Fig. 1. Course of the hypoglossal nerve as it courses distally toward the tongue and its associated musculature. The geniohyoid muscle is innervated by the first cervical nerve branch (C1), which is included for stimulation. GGo/GGh, genioglossus oblique and horizontal components; GH, geniohyoid; HG, hyoglossus; IL, inferior longitudinal segment of the intrinsic tongue muscles; SG, styloglossus; T/V, transverse and vertical segments of the intrinsic tongue muscles. (*From* Heiser, C., Thaler, E., Boon, M., Soose, R. J. & Woodson, B. T. Updates of operative techniques for upper airway stimulation. *The Laryngoscope* 126 Suppl 7, S12-16, https://doi.org/10.1002/lary.26158 (2016); with permission.)

The consequences of repeat periods of hypoxia are thought to be the reasons the disease is associated with cardiovascular disease, including cardiac arrhythmias and stroke.[7–11] Arousals and poor sleep quality lead to excessive daytime sleepiness, a common complaint among OSA patients that is associated with increased accidents in the workplace and motor vehicle accidents.[12,13] There are clear associations between OSA and all-cause morbidity and mortality.[14,15] The pathophysiology of OSA is complex with multiple factors contributing to a balance between a patient's respiratory control, upper airway size, pharyngeal muscle response, and arousability.[16–18]

First-line therapy for OSA is noninvasive continuous positive airway pressure therapy (CPAP).[19] CPAP consists of a pressure-generating machine connected to a face mask. The patient wears the mask during sleep, and positive pressure is applied to stent open the airway during sleep. It is a noninvasive therapy with few side effects; however, adherence to therapy in the population is low with only 40% to 60% of OSA patients ultimately maintaining treatment.[20]

Alternative therapies for treatment of OSA include oral appliances and a variety of surgical techniques, including genioglossus advancement, hyoid suspension, tongue base reduction, adenotonsillectomy, uvulopalatopharyngoplasty, and skeletal advancement surgery.[21–26] A drawback of these surgeries is that they are static procedures, relying on ablation or repositioning of soft tissue in the upper airway without paying attention to the dynamic process by which apnea occurs. As such, surgical therapies have had wide varying levels of success for treatment of OSA. Nerve stimulation is an attractive and novel alternative for treatment of apnea because it helps modify changes in muscular tone and dilator activity that accompany apneic events.

HGNS for treatment of OSA, also known as upper airway stimulation surgery (UAS), targets the genioglossus and portions of the intrinsic tongue musculature. The desired effect is tongue protrusion and stiffening in order to dilate the pharynx to prevent airflow limitation from collapse of the pharyngeal musculature. The genioglossus muscle is the largest dilator of the pharynx and an ideal target for this purpose. Activation of the intrinsic tongue musculature occurs in conjunction to stiffen the tongue to prevent posterior pharyngeal collapse.[3] There is also indirect visual evidence of "palate-glossal coupling," whereby the retropalate opens with nerve stimulation of the tongue musculature because of the interactions of the genioglossus and palatoglossus muscles (**Fig. 2**).[27]

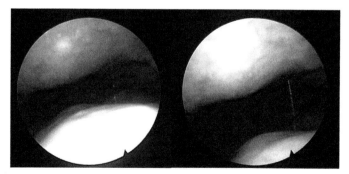

Fig. 2. Endoscopic visualization of the soft palate and posterior pharynx before and after activation of the hypoglossal nerve stimulator in an awake patient. There is an increase in size of the soft palate lumen in association with tongue protrusion from device activation suggestive of "palate-glossal coupling."

Early animal model studies in the late 1980s and early 1990s demonstrated that direct stimulation of the hypoglossal nerve was a viable method of dilating the upper airway, increasing airflow and further decreasing the negative pressure needed to collapse the upper airway.[28,29] At around the same time, attempts at both transcutaneous and direct stimulation of the nerve were being performed in humans. Submental transcutaneous stimulation of the hypoglossal nerve in adult OSA patients did not improve obstructive apneas, but direct stimulation of the genioglossus using fine wire electrodes did show a decrease in frequency of obstructive apneas.[30–32] A decade later, the first prototypes of HGNS implants were being trialed in human volunteers that eventually led to approval of the first UAS device.[33]

Currently, there is only 1 Food and Drug Administration (FDA) -approved UAS device available for the treatment of OSA. Inspire (Inspire Medical Systems, Golden Valley, MN, USA) was FDA approved in 2014.[4] Other devices are currently in development (ImThera Medical, San Diego, CA, USA), but none have been FDA approved as of the writing of this chapter.[34] Because of this, most of the work in UAS will be focused on the function and outcomes of the Inspire implant.

UAS was first FDA approved for the treatment of OSA in 2014. The Stimulation for Apnea Reduction trial was the landmark trial that showed the viability of neurostimulation for the treatment of OSA.[4] One hundred twenty-six patients with OSA were implanted with the Inspire device. Following implantation, patients saw an average reduction of AHI 16.4 events/hr, with 66% of participants achieving surgical success as defined as an AHI reduction of greater than 50% from baseline and an AHI less than 20 events/hr. Patients have been followed since initial implantation, and on 60-month follow-up, patients were shown to have a continued durable response from therapy.[35] More recent postapproval outcomes data from the ADHERE registry, which consists of 508 patients who received UAS implants, showed an overall surgical success rate of 81%.[36] Moreover, average usage of the device was 5.7 hours a night every night compared to CPAP adherence which only ranges from 30% to 60% with a minimum adherence criteria of only 4 hours a night for 5 nights a week.

Epworth Sleepiness Scale (ESS) and Functional Outcomes of Sleep Questionnaire (FOSQ) were recorded patient-reported outcomes measures in the STAR trial. ADHERE registry patients had ESS reported as well. Average ESS and FOSQ showed statistically significant improvements in both subjective sleepiness and quality-of-life outcomes with UAS therapy.[4,36] With regards to patient impressions of the procedure, 94% of ADHERE registry patients reported a better experience with UAS than with CPAP, and 96% of patients would recommend the procedure to a family member or friend. Ultimately, 94% of patients were satisfied with the procedure.[36]

DESCRIPTION OF THE DEVICE

Inspire (Inspire Medical Systems) is currently the only FDA-approved UAS for the treatment of OSA. It works by electrically stimulating the hypoglossal nerve during sleep to dilate and stiffen the upper airway. The device consists of 3 main components: a stimulating electrode, an implantable pulse generator (IPG), and a pressure sensor (**Fig. 3**). The electrode is placed around the hypoglossal nerve. The IPG is placed in a subcutaneous pocket within the chest, overlying the pectoralis major muscle. The pressure sensor is placed between the external and internal intercostal muscles within the chest to detect respirations. During inspiration, the pressure sensor sends a signal to the IPG, which generates an electrical stimulus that is

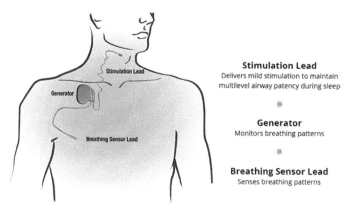

Stimulation Lead
Delivers mild stimulation to maintain
multilevel airway patency during sleep

Generator
Monitors breathing patterns

Breathing Sensor Lead
Senses breathing patterns

Fig. 3. The UAS system with a pulse generator implanted in the right chest connected to a sensor lead going between the intercostal muscles in the chest and a stimulation lead going to the hypoglossal nerve. (*Courtesy of* Inspire Medical Systems, Golden Valley, MN; with permission.)

directed to the stimulating electrode to stimulate the hypoglossal nerve (**Figs. 4** and **5** shows a schematic of sensor and stimulation leads). Stimulation of the nerve, therefore, occurs intermittently in coordination with breathing to dilate the airway during inspiration.

The device is activated via a wireless remote that the patient places over the IPG on the chest to turn on the device before sleep (**Figs. 6–8**). There are adjustable settings for the timing of activation so patients have the option of delaying activation until they fall asleep. The device can also be temporarily paused if the patient awakens in the night. There are also adjustable voltage intensity settings, which are determined after a titration polysomnogram that allow the patient to slowly increase the intensity over several weeks in order to improve tolerance to the electrical stimulus.

The electrode configuration of the stimulating lead consists of a central electrode surrounded on 2 sides by a second electrode. The electrodes are within a flexible self-sizing cuff that is meant to wrap around the hypoglossal nerve without applying significant pressure that may injure the nerve. There is also an electrode built within the IPG. Typically, the central electrode of the stimulating lead serves as the negative

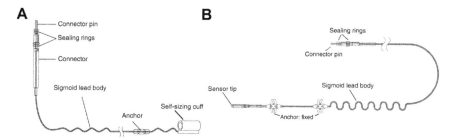

Fig. 4. Stimulation and sensor leads. (*A*) Stimulation lead: the positive and negative electrodes are within the sizing cuff, which is placed around the lateral branches of the hypoglossal nerve, including the C1 branch to the geniohyoid when possible. (*B*) Sensor lead: the distal sensor tip has a pressure-sensitive membrane that responds to the actions of intercostal muscles during inspiration. (*Courtesy of* Inspire Medical Systems, Golden Valley, MN; with permission.)

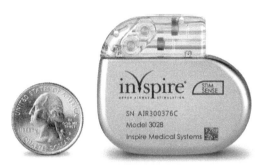

Fig. 5. IPG. (*Courtesy of* Inspire Medical Systems, Golden Valley, MN; with permission.)

pole, and the surrounding electrode is the positive pole. Electrical stimulus is generated between the negative and positive poles. Configuration of the electrodes can be modified. The electrodes can be reversed with the central electrode being positive, and the positive pole surrounded by the negative pole on both sides. The IPG can also serve as the positive pole while maintaining the stimulating lead as the negative pole which directs the electrical signal from the stimulating lead toward the IPG in the chest, creating a more diffuse distribution of the electrical stimulus. Although not commonly adjusted, these settings can help with patient comfort to device stimulation. There is research currently looking into whether different settings may improve outcomes.

The IPG is battery powered and will last an estimated 11 years. Once the battery expires, surgical exposure of the IPG and replacement will be required for continued therapy. The Inspire model 3024 IPG is not MRI compatible, but the new current model 3028 IPG is compatible for MRI of the head and extremities under certain conditions.

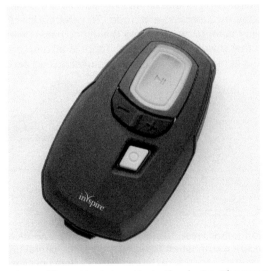

Fig. 6. Wireless remote used by patients to activate the device. The remote is placed on the chest overlying the IPG in order to turn the device on. (*Courtesy of* Inspire Medical Systems, Golden Valley, MN; with permission.)

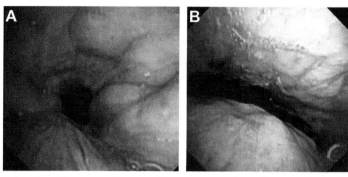

Fig. 7. DISE showing (*A*) concentric versus (*B*) anteroposterior collapse at the level of the soft palate. Studies have shown that patients with concentric collapse at the level of the soft palate do worse with UAS.

PREOPERATIVE WORKUP

UAS is currently approved for patients over the age of 22 with body mass index less than 35 and moderate to severe OSA (AHI between 15 and 65 events per hour) who are unable to tolerate CPAP therapy. An up-to-date polysomnogram should be obtained to confirm the diagnosis of OSA which can either be an in-laboratory polysomnogram or a home sleep apnea test. Patients considering UAS should be evaluated by both a sleep physician and a surgeon qualified to perform UAS implantation. Alternative options should be discussed, including optimizing CPAP therapy, use of bilevel positive airway pressure or other alternative positive airway pressure device, weight loss, positional therapy, alternative surgical procedures, and oral appliance.

Those who are interested in surgery must first undergo drug-induced sleep endoscopy (DISE) to determine if they qualify for UAS surgery. DISE involves intraoperative endoscopic upper airway assessment under controlled sedation that attempts to simulate the upper airway collapse during sleep. Assessment of retropalatal, retroglossal, and supraglottic regions should be assessed during DISE. The presence of anteroposterior collapse at the retropalatal region will qualify for UAS. Patients with

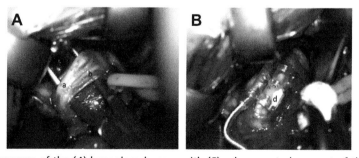

Fig. 8. Exposure of the (*A*) hypoglossal nerve with (*B*) subsequent placement of the stimulation lead electrode around the lateral branches of the hypoglossal nerve. (a) The main hypoglossal nerve trunk as it separates into distal branches. (b) The C1 branch to the geniohyoid, which is included in the cuff. (c) The medial branches of the hypoglossal nerve, which innervate the retractors of the tongue that are excluded from stimulation. (d) The electrode around the lateral branches of the hypoglossal nerve and the C1 branch to the geniohyoid muscle.

concentric collapse at the retropalatal region were shown to be more likely to fail therapy and therefore should not receive UAS (**Table 1**).[37]

Other contraindications listed by the company include the following:

- Central + mixed apneas greater than 25% of the total AHI.
- Any condition or procedure that has compromised neurologic control of the upper airway.
- Patients who are unable or do not have the necessary assistance to operate the sleep remote.
- Patients who are pregnant or plan to become pregnant.
- Patients who are arc welders.

SURGICAL TECHNIQUE

The procedure is performed under general anesthesia. Neuromonitoring of the hypoglossal nerve is performed (ie NIM-Response 3.0 System; Medtronic Xomed, Jacksonville, FL, USA) with placement of electrode leads in the floor of mouth and ipsilateral lateral tongue. These electrodes will record genioglossus and hyoglossus activity, respectively. Neuromonitoring is important because as the hypoglossal nerve branches, inclusion of only the nerve branches feeding the protrusors (genioglossus) of the tongue and exclusion of nerves feeding into the retractors (hyoglossus, styloglossus) of the tongue will ensure maximum tongue protrusion and upper airway dilation on stimulation. Because active stimulation of the tongue will be performed during the procedure, long-acting paralytics should be avoided.

The surgical site includes 3 areas corresponding to the 3 main stages of the procedure. The surgical field starts at the angle of the mandible and extends down to the lower edge of the ribcage between the sternum and the posterior axilla. During surgical preparation, a clear plastic sterile drape is placed from the mandible over the head. The clear drape allows for visualization of the tongue during neurostimulation as well as initial testing of the device immediately after implantation. The implant is typically placed on the right side, although left-sided implantation can be performed if medically required.

The first stage of the procedure is identifying the hypoglossal nerve and placement of the stimulating electrode. A 4-cm incision is made in the ipsilateral upper neck 1 to 2 cm below the inferior border of the mandible. The posterior border of the incision should be just anterior to the submandibular gland and below the mandible to avoid injury to the marginal mandibular nerve. Anteriorly, the midline chin, neck, and thyroid notch are consistent landmarks to identify. Once the incision is made, dissection through the platysma is performed and both the anterior belly of the digastric and the anterior border of the submandibular gland should be identified. The digastric

Table 1	
Summary of requirements for upper airway stimulation candidacy	
Criteria for UAS candidacy	
Minimum age (y)	22
Body mass index	35
AHI	15-65 events/h
Central apneas	<25% of AHI events
DISE	No concentric collapse of the soft palate

muscle is then followed posteriorly to the digastric tendon. Palpation of the hyoid bone can help locate the digastric tendon if exposure is difficult. Exposure of a portion of anterior belly of the digastric muscle is helpful because it improves anterior retraction of the muscle when exposing the hypoglossal nerve. Dissection deep to the posterior border of the anterior belly of the digastric muscle will expose the mylohyoid muscle, which will be bordering the submandibular gland. The anterior portion of the hypoglossal nerve will lie deep to this muscle. Retraction of the submandibular gland posteriorly and the mylohyoid muscle anteriorly will reveal the hypoglossal nerve. Commonly, the nerve is intimately associated with the vena comitans (ranine veins) of the hypoglossal nerve, which follow the nerve and drain into the lingual vein. These veins may need to be controlled and tied in order to expose the nerve without risk of bleeding. As the main branch of the hypoglossal nerve is dissected anteriorly, it will begin to branch. Neurostimulation is important at this time in order to identify branches to the genioglossus and intrinsic tongue musculature, which should be included in the electrode placement for stimulation. Branches to the styloglossus and hyoglossus, which are retractor muscles, should not be included in electrode placement. Once all the inclusion branches are identified, the stimulation electrode is placed around those nerve branches and secured by anchoring the lead to the digastric muscle.

The second stage of the procedure is placement of the impulse generator in the anterior chest. A 4- to 5-cm incision is placed along the ipsilateral chest about 3 cm inferior to the clavicle. Once the incision is made, dissection through the subcutaneous fat is performed until there is exposure of the fascia pectoralis muscle. A pocket overlying the fascia of the pectoralis muscle is then made to accommodate the IPG.

The final stage is placement of the sensor lead within the intercostal muscles of the ribs. This incision is made along the anterior midaxillary line overlying the intercostal space between the fourth and sixth ribs. Preoperative palpation of the ribs can help direct where to place the incision. It is preferable to select the most superior rib space palpable because the inferior rib spaces may be inferior to the diaphragm, making sensation of respirations by the sensing lead more difficult. Once the incision is made, blunt dissection down to the intercostal muscles is performed. The first muscular landmark typically encountered is the serratus anterior muscle, which originates from the scapula and inserts onto the ribs. The serratus anterior muscle should not be confused with the intercostal muscles. After dissection through the serratus anterior, the external intercostal muscle will be identified. Gently dissecting deep to the external intercostals will reveal the internal intercostal muscles. A change in the direction of the muscle fibers will be seen at the transition between external and internal intercostal muscles. Using a malleable retractor, a pocket is made between the internal and external intercostal muscles. The sensor lead is then placed into the pocket and secured to the fascia of the chest. Both the electrode and the sensor lead are then tunneled subcutaneously from their respective sites into the anterior chest incision to connect to the IPG. Before surgical closure, the device is activated to test that the sensor lead is in good position to identify respirations and that the stimulation lead protrudes the tongue. If either of the 2 leads has problems, then revision should be performed before closure.

After closure, pressure dressings are placed over the incisions, and the patient's arm is kept in an arm sling for 72 hours to prevent excessive motion and strain while the implant is healing. The patient is seen at 1 week for a wound check to ensure proper healing. At 1 month after surgery, the device is activated in the clinic for the patient to begin using. After a month of acclimatization to device use and continued healing, a formal titration PSG is performed to determine optimum settings.

COMPLICATION RATES

Serious adverse events were reported in less than 2% of STAR trial participants. Two patients from the study required additional surgical intervention to reposition the neurostimulator for discomfort. Changes to tongue sensation, temporary weakness, and stimulation discomfort were the most common initial complaints. Eighteen percent of participants had temporary tongue weakness; 40% reported discomfort with stimulation, and 21% reported tongue soreness or abrasions related to stimulation. Most symptom complaints resolved within several months with adjustment of device settings.[4]

Adverse events reports from the ADHERE registry showed an intraoperative and immediate postoperative complication rate of 2%. One of the 508 patients (<1%) required revision surgery for a dislodged stimulation lead, which was readjusted without incident. Postoperative adverse events were reported in 23% of patients, most of which were related to discomfort of the implant and/or its stimulation.[36]

FUTURE DIRECTIONS

Although only approved for OSA patients over the age of 22, there are case reports of this device being used in pediatric Down patients as an alternative to CPAP therapy.[38,39] In the future, HGNS will likely have a greater role in the treatment of OSA in the syndromic pediatric population where CPAP may not be tolerated and conventional surgeries are ineffective.

Use of therapy is a major criticism of CPAP therapy. Large studies looking at cardiovascular outcomes of CPAP therapy have failed to show decreased cardiovascular risk from therapy.[11] The lack of cardiovascular response has been partly blamed on the fact that participants on average used CPAP for less than 4 hours a night. One asset of UAS for treatment of OSA is that implanted patients use the device nearly 6 hours a night. There is already research looking at the cardiovascular consequences of UAS, and likely more studies will be seen in the future looking at health outcomes with UAS, which may help further delineate the role OSA plays in cardiovascular and other medical comorbid risks.[40]

UAS for treatment of OSA has an 81% success rate. More research is needed to determine why 19% of patients fail therapy despite rigorous preoperative evaluation and workup. OSA is a complex illness that involves many physiologic factors, including a patient's respiratory control, sleep depth, upper airway size, and pharyngeal muscle response. Further studies looking at how these factors may contribute to UAS success will be important to better select patients for whom the therapy will succeed.

SUMMARY

HGNS is a novel strategy for the treatment of OSA. Its anatomy allows for easy surgical access, and its function as a motor nerve allows for tolerable neurostimulation. It has shown success as a therapy for the treatment of OSA and will likely see more expanded use in a wider population for treatment of OSA. Patients who use the device not only show improvement in symptoms but also tolerate the device well with a large majority preferring it over CPAP therapy. Future studies will look at the effects of UAS on medical outcomes in the treatment of OSA as well as in improving the understanding of the pathophysiology of OSA to better select patients for surgery.

DISCLOSURE

Dr E.R. Thaler has received honorariums from Inspire Medical Systems for speaking at past conferences. Dr J.L. Yu has nothing to disclose.

REFERENCES

1. Bademci G, Yasargil MG. Microsurgical anatomy of the hypoglossal nerve. J Clin Neurosci 2006;13:841–7.
2. Iaconetta G, Solari D, Villa A, et al. The hypoglossal nerve: anatomical study of its entire course. World Neurosurg 2018;109:e486–92.
3. Sanders I, Mu L. A three-dimensional atlas of human tongue muscles. Anat Rec (Hoboken) 2013;296:1102–14.
4. Strollo PJ Jr, Soose RJ, Maurer JT, et al. Upper-airway stimulation for obstructive sleep apnea. N Engl J Med 2014;370:139–49.
5. Peppard PE, Young T, Barnet JH, et al. Increased prevalence of sleep-disordered breathing in adults. Am J Epidemiol 2013;177:1006–14.
6. Berry RB, Budhiraja R, Gottlieb DJ, et al. Rules for scoring respiratory events in sleep: update of the 2007 AASM manual for the scoring of sleep and associated events. Deliberations of the Sleep Apnea Definitions Task Force of the American Academy of Sleep Medicine. J Clin Sleep Med 2012;8:597–619.
7. Wright J, Johns R, Watt I, et al. Health effects of obstructive sleep apnoea and the effectiveness of continuous positive airways pressure: a systematic review of the research evidence. BMJ 1997;314:851–60.
8. Gami AS, Pressman G, Caples SM, et al. Association of atrial fibrillation and obstructive sleep apnea. Circulation 2004;110:364–7.
9. Yaggi HK, Concato J, Kernan WN, et al. Obstructive sleep apnea as a risk factor for stroke and death. N Engl J Med 2005;353:2034–41.
10. Mehra R, Benjamin EJ, Shahar E, et al. Association of nocturnal arrhythmias with sleep-disordered breathing: the Sleep Heart Health Study. Am J Respir Crit Care Med 2006;173:910–6.
11. McEvoy RD, Antic NA, Heeley E, et al. CPAP for prevention of cardiovascular events in obstructive sleep apnea. N Engl J Med 2016;375:919–31.
12. Garbarino S, Guglielmi O, Sanna A, et al. Risk of occupational accidents in workers with obstructive sleep apnea: systematic review and meta-analysis. Sleep 2016;39:1211–8.
13. Tregear S, Reston J, Schoelles K, et al. Obstructive sleep apnea and risk of motor vehicle crash: systematic review and meta-analysis. J Clin Sleep Med 2009;5:573–81.
14. Pan L, Xie X, Liu D, et al. Obstructive sleep apnoea and risks of all-cause mortality: preliminary evidence from prospective cohort studies. Sleep Breath 2016;20:345–53.
15. Fu Y, Xia Y, Yi H, et al. Meta-analysis of all-cause and cardiovascular mortality in obstructive sleep apnea with or without continuous positive airway pressure treatment. Sleep Breath 2017;21:181–9.
16. Remmers JE, deGroot WJ, Sauerland EK, et al. Pathogenesis of upper airway occlusion during sleep. J Appl Physiol Respir Environ Exerc Physiol 1978;44:931–8.
17. Wellman A, Eckert DJ, Jordan AS, et al. A method for measuring and modeling the physiological traits causing obstructive sleep apnea. J Appl Physiol (1985) 2011;110:1627–37.
18. Amatoury J, Azarbarzin A, Younes M, et al. Arousal intensity is a distinct pathophysiological trait in obstructive sleep apnea. Sleep 2016;39:2091–100.
19. Sullivan CE, Issa FG, Berthon-Jones M, et al. Reversal of obstructive sleep apnoea by continuous positive airway pressure applied through the nares. Lancet 1981;1:862–5.

20. Sawyer AM, Gooneratne NS, Marcus CL, et al. A systematic review of CPAP adherence across age groups: clinical and empiric insights for developing CPAP adherence interventions. Sleep Med Rev 2011;15:343–56.
21. Fujita S, Conway W, Zorick F, et al. Surgical correction of anatomic abnormalities in obstructive sleep apnea syndrome: uvulopalatopharyngoplasty. Otolaryngol Head Neck Surg 1981;89:923–34.
22. Johnson NT, Chinn J. Uvulopalatopharyngoplasty and inferior sagittal mandibular osteotomy with genioglossus advancement for treatment of obstructive sleep apnea. Chest 1994;105:278–83.
23. Zaghi S, Holty JE, Certal V, et al. Maxillomandibular advancement for treatment of obstructive sleep apnea: a meta-analysis. JAMA Otolaryngol Head Neck Surg 2016;142:58–66.
24. Holty JE, Guilleminault C. Maxillomandibular advancement for the treatment of obstructive sleep apnea: a systematic review and meta-analysis. Sleep Med Rev 2010;14:287–97.
25. Handler E, Hamans E, Goldberg AN, et al. Tongue suspension: an evidence-based review and comparison to hypopharyngeal surgery for OSA. Laryngoscope 2014;124:329–36.
26. Murphey AW, Kandl JA, Nguyen SA, et al. The effect of glossectomy for obstructive sleep apnea: a systematic review and meta-analysis. Otolaryngol Head Neck Surg 2015;153:334–42.
27. Heiser C, Edenharter G, Bas M, et al. Palatoglossus coupling in selective upper airway stimulation. Laryngoscope 2017;127:E378–83.
28. Miki H, Hida W, Shindoh C, et al. Effects of electrical stimulation of the genioglossus on upper airway resistance in anesthetized dogs. Am Rev Respir Dis 1989;140:1279–84.
29. Schwartz AR, Thut DC, Russ B, et al. Effect of electrical stimulation of the hypoglossal nerve on airflow mechanics in the isolated upper airway. Am Rev Respir Dis 1993;147:1144–50.
30. Edmonds LC, Daniels BK, Stanson AW, et al. The effects of transcutaneous electrical stimulation during wakefulness and sleep in patients with obstructive sleep apnea. Am Rev Respir Dis 1992;146:1030–6.
31. Guilleminault C, Powell N, Bowman B, et al. The effect of electrical stimulation on obstructive sleep apnea syndrome. Chest 1995;107:67–73.
32. Eisele DW, Smith PL, Alam DS, et al. Direct hypoglossal nerve stimulation in obstructive sleep apnea. Arch Otolaryngol Head Neck Surg 1997;123:57–61.
33. Schwartz AR, Bennett ML, Smith PL, et al. Therapeutic electrical stimulation of the hypoglossal nerve in obstructive sleep apnea. Arch Otolaryngol Head Neck Surg 2001;127:1216–23.
34. Friedman M, Jacobowitz O, Hwang MS, et al. Targeted hypoglossal nerve stimulation for the treatment of obstructive sleep apnea: six-month results. Laryngoscope 2016;126:2618–23.
35. Woodson BT, Strohl KP, Soose RJ, et al. Upper airway stimulation for obstructive sleep apnea: 5-year outcomes. Otolaryngol Head Neck Surg 2018;159:194–202.
36. Heiser C, Steffen A, Boon M, et al. Post-approval upper airway stimulation predictors of treatment effectiveness in the ADHERE registry. Eur Respir J 2019;53. https://doi.org/10.1183/13993003.01405-2018.
37. Vanderveken OM, Maurer JT, Hohenhorst W, et al. Evaluation of drug-induced sleep endoscopy as a patient selection tool for implanted upper airway stimulation for obstructive sleep apnea. J Clin Sleep Med 2013;9:433–8.

38. Diercks GR, Keamy D, Kinane TB, et al. Hypoglossal nerve stimulator implantation in an adolescent with Down syndrome and sleep apnea. Pediatrics 2016; 137. https://doi.org/10.1542/peds.2015-3663.
39. Diercks GR, Wentland C, Keamy D, et al. Hypoglossal nerve stimulation in adolescents with Down syndrome and obstructive sleep apnea. JAMA Otolaryngol Head Neck Surg 2017. https://doi.org/10.1001/jamaoto.2017.1871.
40. Dedhia RC, Shah AJ, Bliwise DL, et al. Hypoglossal nerve stimulation and heart rate variability: analysis of STAR trial responders. Otolaryngol Head Neck Surg 2019;160:165–71.

Light-Based Neuronal Activation

The Future of Cranial Nerve Stimulation

Elliott D. Kozin, MD*, M. Christian Brown, PhD, Daniel J. Lee, MD,
Konstantina M. Stankovic, MD, PhD

KEYWORDS

- Infrared neural stimulation • Optogenetics • Opsins

KEY POINTS

- Electrical neuronal stimulation has inherent limitations, including nonspecific current spread and electrode channel crosstalk.
- Light-based stimulation offers a theoretical advantage over electrical stimulation because it may allow for improved spatial selectivity.
- The two major light-based stimulation paradigms include infrared and optogenetic neural stimulation.
- Optogenetic neuronal stimulation requires genetic modification of neurons and delivery of opsin genes that encode for light-gated transmembrane ions channels.
- Future applications for optogenetic technology include cochlear implants, auditory brainstem implants, retinal implants, and facial nerve implants.

OVERVIEW

Biomedical devices that electrically stimulate cranial nerves, such as the cochlear implant (CI), have had widespread worldwide success. However, despite advances in neuroprosthetic implant hardware and software, devices have sustained evolutionary rather than revolutionary changes. The outcome ceiling of neuroprosthetic implants is partly due to properties of electricity stimulation. Electrical therapy dates back nearly 2000 years, when Scribonius Largus used electrical shocks from a live black torpedo fish for electrotherapy to provide relief for a variety of symptoms, including pain and gout.[1] Centuries later, Galvani stimulated the cochleovestibular nerve in the 1790s, and pacemakers, CIs, and deep brain stimulators followed in the late twentieth century.[2] Today, more advanced electrically based biomedical

Massachusetts Eye and Ear Infirmary and Harvard Medical School, 243 Charles Street, Boston, MA 02114, USA
* Corresponding author.
E-mail address: Elliott_Kozin@meei.harvard.edu

Otolaryngol Clin N Am 53 (2020) 171–183
https://doi.org/10.1016/j.otc.2019.09.011
0030-6665/20/© 2019 Elsevier Inc. All rights reserved.

devices all used electrodes to generate a charge near a nerve cell to open electrically gated ion channels of neurons.

Building on the success of current implant technology, researchers have identified key characteristics of neuroprosthetics. The ideal neuroprosthetic has fast temporal and precise spatial resolution that is able to depolarize a neuron quickly and specifically. Although electrical stimulation provides the capacity for fast temporal resolution, it has limited spatial selectivity. Nonspecific electrical stimulation results in unwanted current spread and channel crosstalk, potentially limiting outcomes and generating side effects.[3–5] In addition, overlapping current fields from different electrodes or channel interaction in multichannel electrode arrays may reduce the number of effective channels available for transmitting information.[6,7]

As an example of limitations of electrical stimulation, hearing outcomes of the CI are variable across similar patient cohorts,[8,9] and CI users have deficits in understanding speech in noisy environments[10–13] and in musical appreciation.[14] CIs can also result in unwanted stimulation, such as facial nerve stimulation.[15] One approach to improving outcomes of CIs has been to increase the number of electrode channels, which would theoretically improve spatial resolution. Unfortunately, studies have illustrated that the number of useful channels in the CI is small, typically fewer than 10.[11] This situation arises because each channel broadly activates spiral ganglion neurons (SGN). Adding additional channels does not activate discrete populations of SGNs.[16]

Alternative strategies for neuronal stimulation are currently being investigated with the primary goal of improving spatial selectivity. The most promising alternative strategy is light-based neuronal activation. Light-based stimulation offers a theoretic advantage over electric-based stimulation because it can target specific neurons, increasing the number of independent stimulation channels while reducing the unintended consequence of current spread.[10,17] Thus, the ability to harness light to depolarize neurons could increase the spatial resolution of implants and offer more independent channels, thereby improving implant outcomes.

In this article, we provide a broad overview of two light-based neuronal stimulation paradigms: infrared neural stimulation (INS) and optogenetic neural stimulation (ONS). In addition, we provide examples of light-based prostheses, including CIs, auditory brainstem implants, retinal implants, and facial nerve implants. The article concludes with future directions for electrical and light-based neurostimulation.

INFRARED AND OPTOGENETIC NEURAL STIMULATION

INS and ONS have fundamentally different approaches to neuronal activation. INS uses light from the infrared spectrum to stimulate unmodified neurons. In contrast, optogenetics uses light from various wavelengths within the visible spectrum to stimulate modified neurons that have been altered by gene transfer to gain light sensitivity (**Table 1**). In the following section, we discuss basic principles of INS and ONS.

Infrared Neural Stimulation

INS uses infrared wavelengths of light to cause neuronal excitation. Several studies have demonstrated that INS can stimulate peripheral nerves, cortical neurons, and muscles.[18] INS may be applied to any neuron, whereas optogenetics requires genetic modification of specific neurons to render them sensitive to light. Thus, a theoretic advantage of INS is the ability to stimulate neurons without genetic manipulation of target tissues. Studies have indicated that infrared light is capable of depolarizing unmodified neurons with significantly less spread of neural activation compared with

Table 1
Definitions

Term	Definition
Infrared neural stimulation	Pulses of infrared light are delivered to the neural tissue to control cellular events.
Optogenetics	Biomedical technique that uses light to control cells, which have been modified to express light-sensitive ion channels.
Opsin	Light-gated transmembrane ion channel.
Electrode	Conductor through which electricity is transmitted to target tissue (eg, neurons).
Optrode	Conductor through which light is transmitted to target tissue (eg, neurons).

electrical stimulation.[1] It is theorized that INS results in neuronal action potentials because of thermal gradients.[18]

Several studies have examined the use of INS to stimulate the peripheral auditory system in a variety of in vivo models.[19–27] There are several aspects of INS, however, that may affect translation into the clinic. Infrared light generates thermal gradients to depolarize neurons, which results in heat that may potentially be harmful to tissues.[7,28,29] Moreover, the energy required for INS may exceed what is currently practical for use in portable prostheses.[30]

Studies have also demonstrated that optoacoustic artifacts may confound INS findings in peripheral[31] and central auditory systems.[32] Some studies using INS to stimulate the auditory system have failed to elicit auditory responses in deafened animal models.[33,34] However, more recent studies are beginning to address potential mechanisms of INS stimulation in deafened animal models and applicability to modifying electrically based neuronal stimulation.[24] Thus, although INS may not be a viable stand-alone option for neuronal stimulation at the current time, its ability to modulate neurons may provide exciting avenues for clinical utility.

Optogenetics

Optogenetics refers to the use of optics and genetics to control neuronal action potentials (see **Table 1**).[35] Optogenetic technology is based on opsins, which are light-sensitive proteins that can control cellular events. In an ONS paradigm, opsins are delivered to neurons using contemporary gene transfer techniques. On stimulation with a specific wavelength of light, only neurons that express the light-sensitive opsin will respond. This type of specific neuronal stimulation differs significantly from an electric-based stimulation paradigm, which is generally nonspecific (**Fig. 1**). Most opsins respond to visible wavelengths of light, which limits issues related to unwanted tissue heating.

Classic opsins are light-gated transmembrane ions channel and are categorized into microbial-type (type I) and mammalian-type (type II) opsins. Photons (light) are absorbed by the opsin protein, which subsequently changes conformation. Structural changes to a central pore allow cation entry into the cell resulting in depolarization. Type I opsin genes are the primary type of opsin used by neuroscience laboratories. There are four main categories of type I opsins: (1) bacteriorhodopsin, (2) proteorhodopsin, (3) sensory rhodopsin, and (4) channelrhodopsin (ChR).[34,35] ChR and its variants are the basis of ongoing research using optogenetic technology for neuronal implants. ChR is a light-gated, seven-transmembrane ion channel that was identified in *Chlamydomonas reinhardtii*, a green unicellular algae. The light-sensitive ChR

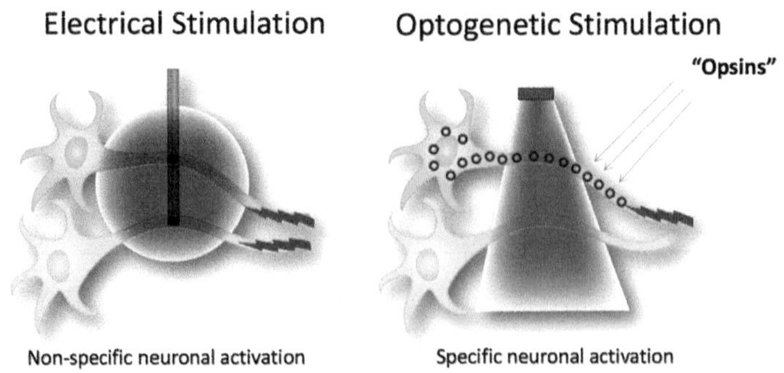

Electrical Stimulation   Optogenetic Stimulation

"Opsins"

Non-specific neuronal activation   Specific neuronal activation

Fig. 1. Nonspecific electrical stimulation versus optogenetic stimulation paradigms. In electrical stimulation, there is broad excitation of many neurons in the vicinity of the electrode (*left*). In optogenetic stimulation, only cells that express opsins and are in the light path are excited (*right*). (*Adapted from* Deisseroth K. Optogenetics. Nat Methods 2011; 8:26-29; with permission.)

transmembrane ion channel opens to allow cellular sodium ion influx on stimulation by light in the blue wavelength. ChR2, a variant of ChR, can sustain control of action potentials in mammalian neurons on the timescale of milliseconds, which is similar to electrical stimulation.[36] ChR2 is now a commonly used opsin for auditory studies (discussed later). Moreover, as optogenetics has expanded, there is a wide array of genetically engineered opsins, varying by light wavelength sensitivity and kinetic properties that can be selected based on desired features (**Fig. 2**).[37]

A key feature of optogenetic neuronal control is the requirement for opsins to be genetically expressed in specific neurons desired for light-dependent activation. Today, optogenetic research relies on (1). transgenic animal lines that express opsins in specific cell types or (2). gene transfer technology to deliver opsin genes to target cells. Opsin-expressing transgenic murine lines are commercially available and readily generated.[38] Although the transgenic approach is commonly used in the laboratory, it is not directly translatable to human studies.

Fortunately, the gene transfer approach is translatable to human studies. Genes may be introduced that provide sensitivity to light. Major translational approaches to delivery of opsins include adenoassociated viral vectors (AAV), lentiviral vectors

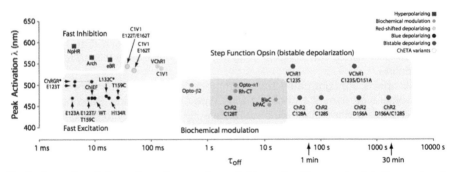

Fig. 2. Examples of the variety of currently available opsins. The graph plots the peak activation wavelength of light as a function of the time constant for a variety of opsins. (*Modified from* Yizhar O, Fenno LE, Davidson TJ, Mogri M, Deisseroth K. Optogenetics in neural systems. Neuron 2011; 71:9-34; with permission.)

(LV), and stems cells. AAV and LV have been applied in a host of mammalian models.[35] LV may be created using standard tissue culture techniques; however, AAV production requires a dedicated vector core, requiring additional resources. Generally, AAV are considered safer than LV because AAV does not broadly integrate into the host genome.

The directed delivery of opsins to specific cells depends on factors beyond the viral packaging and serotype. For example, opsins may be delivered locally, such as via a direct injection, or systemically, such as intravenously. Whether delivered directly or systemically, cellular tropism for certain viral vectors scan help target-specific neuronal cell types and also limit broad expression. In addition to choosing specific viral serotypes that may be more readily transduced in certain cells, tissue-specific promoters may be used. A promoter is a region of DNA that initiates transcription of a particular gene, such as an opsin gene; such promoters may be either broadly expressed or highly tissue specific. By combining a host of different variables, such as choice of opsin, viral vector, tissue-specific promotor, and delivery mechanism, optogenetic models can make specific cell types sensitive to light.

EXAMPLES OF PROSTHESES THAT COULD USE OPTOGENETIC STIMULATION

In the following section, we highlight several ongoing areas of research that are using optogenetic technology for light-based stimulation of cranial nerves. We particularly highlight the CI, auditory brainstem implant (ABI), retinal implant, and facial nerve implant.

Optogenetic-Based Stimulation of the Peripheral Auditory Pathway

The CI is among the most successful of neuroprostheses. CI technology has evolved from a single-channel device to a multichannel auditory neurostimulator providing meaningful speech perception to individuals with severe to profound hearing loss. Despite improvements in technology over the past half-century, auditory neuroprostheses have limitations, especially in noisy environments and in the appreciation of music. Studies from the Massachusetts Eye and Ear,[32,39–42] and the University Medical Center Göttingen,[18,43–47] have illustrated potential for optogenetic technology to overcome current auditory neuroprosthetic limitations. Indeed, optogenetic stimulation has been theorized as a viable option to activate a smaller subset of SGN in the spatially restricted bony modiolus compared with electrical stimulation (**Fig. 3**).[44]

Initial studies of optogenetics in auditory research focused on employing ChR2 in rodent models. In a pioneering paper, Hernandez et al.[44] employed transgenic model and gene therapy murine models to characterize optogenetic stimulation. Optogenetic stimulation of SGNs activated the auditory pathway was measured by single neuron recordings and neuronal population responses. The authors concluded that their study provided a strategy for optogenetic stimulation of the auditory pathway.

Improved spatial resolution has been the primary driver of development of an optogenetic-based neuroprosthetic. Dieter and colleagues[43] successfully tested spectral capacity of optogenetic technology in the peripheral auditory pathway. A gerbil model was used to compare the spectral selectivity of optogenetic, electric, and acoustic stimulation. Investigators found that optogenetic stimulation outperformed bipolar electrical simulation and is not distinguishable from acoustic stimulation at modest intensities. The authors concluded that optogenetics seems to have better spectral selectivity compared with electric SGN stimulation.

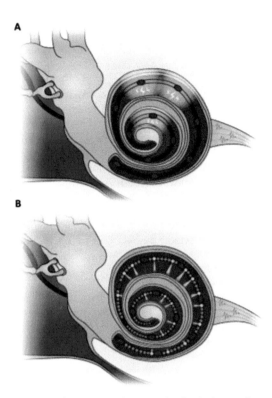

Fig. 3. Schematic overview of optogenetic control of spiral ganglion neurons. This schematic shows a traditional electrical cochlear implant, with broad fields of activation (*A*), and optical cochlear implant, with narrow fields (*B*), which allows for increasing the number of effective channels. (*From* Jeschke M, Moser T. Considering optogenetic stimulation for cochlear implants. Hear Res 2015; 322:224-234; with permission.)

Although improving spatial resolution is a key motivator for optogenetics research, fast temporal resolution is necessary to encode auditory percepts. Unfortunately, ChR2, the classic opsin used in most neuroscience research, has temporal kinetics that allow responses up to a limit, typically less than 100 Hz, well less than temporal properties of a CI.[36,39,48] In the peripheral auditory pathway, Keppeler and colleagues[45] characterized the fast channel rhodopsin, "Chronos."[49] Investigators used a murine AAV model of gene transfer to sensitize SGN to light in the postnatal period. Following transduction of SGNs, fiber-based optical stimulation elicited optical auditory brainstem responses with temporal resolution higher than ChR2. The authors concluded that Chronos may achieve "ultrafast" optogenetic control of SGNs.

In addition to spectral and temporal resolution, efficient gene transfer is a critical aspect on the pathway to clinical translation. Recently, Duarte and colleagues[40] used a novel "ancestral" adenoassociated virus (Anc80) for delivery of opsins to SGNs. Neonatal mice were injected via the round window of cochlea with the specially developed Anc80 vector carrying an opsin (**Fig. 4**). Following an incubation period, pulsed blue light was delivered to cochlear SGNs via a cochleostomy. Optically evoked auditory brainstem responses and multiunit activity in inferior colliculus were

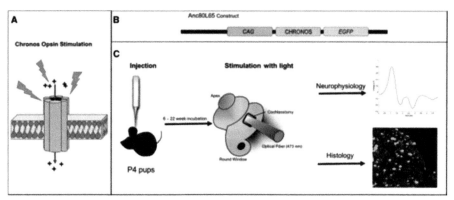

Fig. 4. Methodology for cochlear optogenetics in a murine model. (*A*) Chronos is an ultra-fast light-gated transmembrane ion channel that opens with blue-light stimulation. (*B*) Example of Anc80 construct with a promoter (CAG), opsin (Chronos), and reporter gene (eGFP). (*C*) A murine model for optogenetic injection, blue-light stimulation, neurophysiologic testing via optically evoked potentials, and histology. (*From* Duarte MJ, Kanumuri VV, Landegger LD et al. Ancestral Adeno-Associated Virus Vector Delivery of Opsins to Spiral Ganglion Neurons: Implications for Optogenetic Cochlear Implants. Mol Ther 2018; 26:1931-1939; with permission.)

observed in response to light pulses. Cochlear histology demonstrated robust opsin expression in SGNs with a distribution of the opsin throughout all turns of the cochlea. Duarte and colleagues[40] concluded that the study was the first to describe robust SGN transduction, opsin expression, and optically evoked auditory electrophysiology in neonatal mice.

Optogenetic-Based Stimulation of the Central Auditory Pathway

In addition to investigating optogenetic control of the peripheral auditory system, investigators have also demonstrated stimulation of the central auditory pathway in models of the ABI[39,41,42,50] and auditory midbrain implant.[51] The ABI provides meaningful hearing perception to individuals who cannot benefit from a CI because of anatomic constraints, such as in pediatric patients with cochlear nerve aplasia.[52] Although the CI stimulates SGN of the cochlea, the ABI bypasses a damaged or absent cochlea and/or cochlear nerve to stimulate neurons within the cochlear nucleus (CN).[53,54]

Several landmark in vivo studies have demonstrated the utility of optogenetics in the CN. Shimano and colleagues[50] first demonstrated that ChR2 expression in the CN could activate auditory neurons in a rat model. Using an AAV vector, ChR2 was expressed in all layers of the dorsal subdivision of the CN, which contains second-order auditory neurons. After surgical craniotomy and exposure of the CN, blue light stimulation produced sustained activity in the CN neurons. The opsin expression, as measured by acoustic thresholds, did not impact responses to sound.

Investigators have also developed a murine optogenetic ABI model[39,41,42] based on gene transfer techniques to deliver opsins to the CN.[42] In a subsequent study, Darrow and colleagues[39] demonstrated optically evoked potentials by optogenetic control of CN neurons using pulsed blue light delivered by an optical fiber. In addition, multiunit activity could be directly recorded during these same experiments from the inferior colliculus. Importantly, no optically induced responses were detected in sham-injected mice, ruling out an optoacoustic artifact.

Similar to peripheral studies, investigators have also been able to deliver "ultrafast" opsins, such as Chronos, to the central auditory pathway. In one study, viral-mediated gene transfer for direct injection into the CN was made via a posterolateral craniotomy to express Chronos or ChR2 in the murine model.[41] Following an incubation period after virally mediated gene delivery, blue light was delivered via an optical fiber placed directly on the surface of the CN. Neural activity was recorded in the contralateral inferior colliculus (**Fig. 5**). Both ChR2 and Chronos evoked sustained responses to all stimuli, even at high pulse rates. Synchrony of the light-evoked response to stimulus rates was higher in Chronos compared with ChR2 mice. Thus, Chronos has the ability to drive the auditory system at higher stimulation rates than ChR2 and may be a more ideal opsin for manipulation of auditory pathways.

Behavioral studies in the central auditory pathway using optogenetics have also been completed. Guo and colleagues[8] created an optogenetic murine model of an auditory midbrain implant. Mice were trained to perform an avoidance task based on auditory stimulation. An optic fiber was then implanted into the photosensitized midbrain and the detection task was repeated with photostimulation. In neurophysiologic and behavioral experiments, responses showed that the trained mice were able to "hear the light."

Taken together, research on the development of an optical auditory implant has illustrated feasibility to stimulate the auditory pathway. Ongoing research has focused on generating chronic models of optogenetic stimulation, developing improved gene

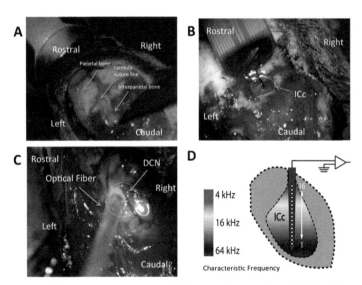

Fig. 5. Mouse model of optogenetic control of the cochlear nucleus. (*A*) The skin and muscle are retracted laterally to expose the cranial suture lines. (*B*) Multielectrode recording probe is placed into the right inferior colliculus. (*C*) Left-sided craniotomy and partial cerebellar aspiration is used to expose the dorsal division of the CN (DCN). An optical fiber is introduced through the craniotomy and onto the CN surface. (*D*) Schematic representation of the recording probe positioned along the tonotopic axis of the inferior colliculus. ICc, central nucleus of the inferior colliculus. (*From* Hight AE, Kozin ED, Darrow Ket al. Superior temporal resolution of Chronos versus channelrhodopsin-2 in an optogenetic model of the auditory brainstem implant. Hear Res 2015; 322:235-241; with permission.)

delivery techniques, optimizing optically based hardware, and determining the ideal "auditory opsin." As gene delivery techniques advance, optogenetic technology may be a viable option in humans.

Optogenetic-Based Retinal Implant

Retinal implants were among the earliest to incorporate optogenetic technology.[2] Bionic solutions to blindness, similar to hearing loss, have been considered for decades. Most classic approaches used electrical stimulation and have necessitated surgical placement of a retinal prosthesis.[2] Surgical placement has potential morbidity on surrounding tissue, and a burdensome cost. In an optogenetic model, an injection containing an opsin could be made to sensitize the retina to light. The individual may then be given a headset to transmit light at appropriate wavelengths.

Among the earliest attempts at an optogenetic retinal prosthesis, Bi and colleagues[55] transfected mouse retinas with ChR2. They found retina-wide expression and were able to elicit evoked potentials in the cortex. Other groups have achieved similar results in various models of retinal degeneration. For example, one Japanese group used ChR2 in a mouse model of retinitis pigmentosa as the basis of visual restoration.[56–58] When transduced on retinal ganglion cells, ChR2 restored visual responses. Optogenetic approaches to the retinal implant are thus a favorable approach to restoring vision in humans.

Optogenetic-Based Facial Nerve Implant

Facial palsy is a devastating condition with functional, emotional, aesthetic, and communication sequelae. Facial nerve paralysis occurs in approximately 40,000 individuals in the United States annually. Currently, there are a variety of options for facial nerve rehabilitation, including medical, physical, and surgical. Unfortunately, dynamic reanimation is limited to smile restoration through nerve or functional muscle transfers. Microelectrode array implantation based on electrical stimulation of the facial nerve has been proposed as an alternative approach (**Fig. 6**).[59] However, current spread may limit the ability to activate discrete facial nerve branches. Current studies are ongoing in a murine whisker movement model to determine if optogenetic technology may address limitations in current electrically based stimulation paradigms.[60]

LIMITATIONS OF OPTOGENETIC TECHNOLOGY AND FUTURE DIRECTIONS

There remain several hurdles before going forward with light-based neuronal stimulation in humans. For INS, ongoing work aims to clarify safety of action and potential optoacoustic artifacts before clinical translation. For optogenetics, there remain several hurdles related to gene transfer techniques and optically based hardware. First, neurons need to be modified to become light sensitive. Neuronal modification requires a host of different factors, including selection of gene transfer techniques and optimized opsins. Future work is needed to optimize the long-term safety and efficacy of gene therapy. Indeed, long-term toxicity of opsins in neurons, such as SGNs, remains unknown. Second, contemporary device hardware is based on electrical stimulation. Light-based stimulation necessitates development of new hardware, which needs to have similar size device footprint and power requirements. For example, current hardware uses electrodes for neuronal stimulation. Multichannel "optrode" arrays may be necessary for optical stimulation. Ultimately, light-based stimulation needs to be demonstrated as being superior to electrically based stimulation.

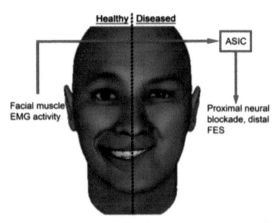

Fig. 6. Neuroprosthetic device for hemifacial reanimation. In an electrical stimulation model, electrode arrays record electromyography (EMG) signals on the healthy side of the face, which then serve as an input for the diseased side. A functional electrical stimulation (FES) control algorithm in an application-specific integrated circuit (ASIC) is used to stimulate distally on the contralateral diseased side. A similar light-based stimulation may potentially allow for improved spatial stimulation of individual branches of the facial nerve. (*From* Jowett N, Kearney RE, Knox CJ, Hadlock TA. Toward the Bionic Face: A Novel Neuroprosthetic Device Paradigm for Facial Reanimation Consisting of Neural Blockade and Functional Electrical Stimulation. Plast Reconstr Surg 2019; 143:62e-76e; with permission.)

In parallel with light-based approaches, improvements to electrical stimulation are also being made. Although outside the scope of this article, there are new areas of research in flexible electrode arrays,[61–65] new electrode contacts,[66] and piezoelectric nanomaterials.[67] In an exciting area of electrical stimulation, piezoelectric materials are able to generate an electric current by mechanical deformation. One could imagine a CI that was powered by fluid oscillations of the basilar membrane of the cochlea, leading to depolarization of hair cells and/or SGN. Early studies have demonstrated proof of concept of the use of these materials in the inner ear.[67] With advances in electrical stimulation and the emerging use of optogenetics, there is an exciting road ahead for neuroprosthetic technology in otolaryngology.

DISCLOSURE

None.

REFERENCES

1. Nutton V. Scribonius Largus, the unknown pharmacologist. Pharm Hist (Lond) 1995;25:5–8.

2. Barrett JM, Berlinguer-Palmini R, Degenaar P. Optogenetic approaches to retinal prosthesis. Vis Neurosci 2014;31:345–54.

3. Boëx C, de Balthasar C, Kos M-I, et al. Electrical field interactions in different cochlear implant systems. J Acoust Soc Am 2003;114:2049.

4. Karg S, Lackner C, Hemmert W. Temporal interaction in electrical hearing elucidates auditory nerve dynamics in humans. Hear Res 2013;299:10–8.

5. Qazi O, van Dijk B, Moonen M, et al. Understanding the effect of noise on electrical stimulation sequences in cochlear implants and its impact on speech intelligibility. Hear Res 2013;299:79–87.
6. Wells J, Kao C, Mariappan K, et al. Optical stimulation of neural tissue in vivo. Opt Lett 2005;30:504–6.
7. Richter CP, Tan X. Photons and neurons. Hear Res 2014;311:72–88.
8. Semenov YR, Martinez-Monedero R, Niparko JK. Cochlear implants: clinical and societal outcomes. Otolaryngol Clin North Am 2012;45:959–81.
9. Ray J, Wright T, Fielden C, et al. Non-users and limited users of cochlear implants. Cochlear Implants Int 2006;7:49–58.
10. Fu QJ, Nogaki G. Noise susceptibility of cochlear implant users: the role of spectral resolution and smearing. J Assoc Res Otolaryngol 2005;6:19–27.
11. Friesen LM, Shannon RV, Baskent D, et al. Speech recognition in noise as a function of the number of spectral channels: comparison of acoustic hearing and cochlear implants. J Acoust Soc Am 2001;110:1150–63.
12. Van Deun L, van Wieringen A, Wouters J. Spatial speech perception benefits in young children with normal hearing and cochlear implants. Ear Hear 2010;31:702–13.
13. Eskridge EN, Galvin JJ 3rd, Aronoff JM, et al. Speech perception with music maskers by cochlear implant users and normal-hearing listeners. J Speech Lang Hear Res 2012;55:800–10.
14. Kohlberg G, Spitzer JB, Mancuso D, et al. Does cochlear implantation restore music appreciation? Laryngoscope 2014;124:587–8.
15. Pires JS, Melo AS, Caiado R, et al. Facial nerve stimulation after cochlear implantation: our experience in 448 adult patients. Cochlear Implants Int 2018;19:193–7.
16. Eisen MD, Franck KH. Electrode interaction in pediatric cochlear implant subjects. J Assoc Res Otolaryngol 2005;6:160–70.
17. Fu QJ, Shannon RV, Wang X. Effects of noise and spectral resolution on vowel and consonant recognition: acoustic and electric hearing. J Acoust Soc Am 1998;104:3586–96.
18. Jeschke M, Moser T. Considering optogenetic stimulation for cochlear implants. Hear Res 2015;322:224–34.
19. Kadakia S, Young H, Richter CP. Masking of infrared neural stimulation (INS) in hearing and deaf guinea pigs. Proc SPIE Int Soc Opt Eng 2013;8565:85655V.
20. Matic AI, Robinson AM, Young HK, et al. Behavioral and electrophysiological responses evoked by chronic infrared neural stimulation of the cochlea. PLoS One 2013;8:e58189.
21. Moreno LE, Rajguru SM, Matic AI, et al. Infrared neural stimulation: beam path in the guinea pig cochlea. Hear Res 2011;282:289–302.
22. Richter CP, Rajguru S, Bendett M. Infrared neural stimulation in the cochlea. Proc SPIE Int Soc Opt Eng 2013;8565:85651Y.
23. Richter CP, Young H. Responses to amplitude modulated infrared stimuli in the guinea pig inferior colliculus. Proc SPIE Int Soc Opt Eng 2013;8656:85655U.
24. Tan X, Jahan I, Xu Y, et al. Auditory neural activity in congenitally deaf mice induced by infrared neural stimulation. Sci Rep 2018;8:388.
25. Tan X, Rajguru S, Young H, et al. Radiant energy required for infrared neural stimulation. Sci Rep 2015;5:13273.
26. Xia N, Tan X, Xu Y, et al. Pressure in the cochlea during infrared irradiation. IEEE Trans Biomed Eng 2018;65:1575–84.
27. Young HK, Tan X, Xia N, et al. Target structures for cochlear infrared neural stimulation. Neurophotonics 2015;2:025002.

28. Wells J, Kao C, Konrad P, et al. Biophysical mechanisms of transient optical stimulation of peripheral nerve. Biophys J 2007;93:2567–80.
29. Wells JD, Thomsen S, Whitaker P, et al. Optically mediated nerve stimulation: identification of injury thresholds. Lasers Surg Med 2007;39:513–26.
30. Richter CP, Rajguru SM, Matic AI, et al. Spread of cochlear excitation during stimulation with pulsed infrared radiation: inferior colliculus measurements. J Neural Eng 2011;8:056006.
31. Teudt IU, Maier H, Richter CP, et al. Acoustic events and "optophonic" cochlear responses induced by pulsed near-infrared laser. IEEE Trans Biomed Eng 2011;58:1648–55.
32. Verma RU, Guex AA, Hancock KE, et al. Auditory responses to electric and infrared neural stimulation of the rat cochlear nucleus. Hear Res 2014;310:69–75.
33. Thompson AC, Fallon JB, Wise AK, et al. Infrared neural stimulation fails to evoke neural activity in the deaf guinea pig cochlea. Hear Res 2015;324:46–53.
34. Fenno L, Yizhar O, Deisseroth K. The development and application of optogenetics. Annu Rev Neurosci 2011;34:389–412.
35. Yizhar O, Fenno LE, Davidson TJ, et al. Optogenetics in neural systems. Neuron 2011;71:9–34.
36. Boyden ES, Zhang F, Bamberg E, et al. Millisecond-timescale, genetically targeted optical control of neural activity. Nat Neurosci 2005;8:1263–8.
37. Deisseroth K. Optogenetics. Nat Methods 2011;8:26–9.
38. Zeng H, Madisen L. Mouse transgenic approaches in optogenetics. Prog Brain Res 2012;196:193–213.
39. Darrow KN, Slama MC, Kozin ED, et al. Optogenetic stimulation of the cochlear nucleus using channelrhodopsin-2 evokes activity in the central auditory pathways. Brain Res 2015;1599:44–56.
40. Duarte MJ, Kanumuri VV, Landegger LD, et al. Ancestral adeno-associated virus vector delivery of opsins to spiral ganglion neurons: implications for optogenetic cochlear implants. Mol Ther 2018;26:1931–9.
41. Hight AE, Kozin ED, Darrow K, et al. Superior temporal resolution of Chronos versus channelrhodopsin-2 in an optogenetic model of the auditory brainstem implant. Hear Res 2015;322:235–41.
42. Kozin ED, Darrow KN, Hight AE, et al. Direct visualization of the murine dorsal cochlear nucleus for optogenetic stimulation of the auditory pathway. J Vis Exp 2015;(95):52426.
43. Dieter A, Duque-Afonso CJ, Rankovic V, et al. Near physiological spectral selectivity of cochlear optogenetics. Nat Commun 2019;10:1962.
44. Hernandez VH, Gehrt A, Reuter K, et al. Optogenetic stimulation of the auditory pathway. J Clin Invest 2014;124:1114–29.
45. Keppeler D, Merino RM, Lopez de la Morena D, et al. Ultrafast optogenetic stimulation of the auditory pathway by targeting-optimized Chronos. EMBO J 2018;37.
46. Scheller D, Durmuller N, Moser P, et al. Continuous stimulation of dopaminergic receptors by rotigotine does not interfere with the sleep-wake cycle in the rat. Eur J Pharmacol 2008;584:111–7.
47. Wrobel C, Dieter A, Huet A, et al. Optogenetic stimulation of cochlear neurons activates the auditory pathway and restores auditory-driven behavior in deaf adult gerbils. Sci Transl Med 2018;10:322–33.
48. Zhang F, Wang LP, Boyden ES, et al. Channelrhodopsin-2 and optical control of excitable cells. Nat Methods 2006;3:785–92.

49. Klapoetke NC, Murata Y, Kim SS, et al. Independent optical excitation of distinct neural populations. Nat Methods 2014;11:338–46.
50. Shimano T, Fyk-Kolodziej B, Mirza N, et al. Assessment of the AAV-mediated expression of channelrhodopsin-2 and halorhodopsin in brainstem neurons mediating auditory signaling. Brain Res 2013;1511:138–52.
51. Guo W, Hight AE, Chen JX, et al. Hearing the light: neural and perceptual encoding of optogenetic stimulation in the central auditory pathway. Sci Rep 2015;5: 10319.
52. Noij KS, Kozin ED, Sethi R, et al. Systematic review of nontumor pediatric auditory brainstem implant outcomes. Otolaryngol Head Neck Surg 2015;153(5):739–50.
53. Hitselberger W, House W, Edgerton B, et al. Cochlear nucleus implant. Otolaryngol Head Neck Surg 1984;92:52–4.
54. Sennaroglu L, Ziyal I, Atas A, et al. Preliminary results of auditory brainstem implantation in prelingually deaf children with inner ear malformations including severe stenosis of the cochlear aperture and aplasia of the cochlear nerve. Otol Neurotol 2009;30:708–15.
55. Bi A, Cui J, Ma YP, et al. Ectopic expression of a microbial-type rhodopsin restores visual responses in mice with photoreceptor degeneration. Neuron 2006; 50:23–33.
56. Tomita H, Sugano E, Yawo H, et al. Restoration of visual response in aged dystrophic RCS rats using AAV-mediated channelopsin-2 gene transfer. Invest Ophthalmol Vis Sci 2007;48:3821–6.
57. Tomita H, Sugano E, Isago H, et al. Channelrhodopsins provide a breakthrough insight into strategies for curing blindness. J Genet 2009;88:409–15.
58. Tomita H, Sugano E, Isago H, et al. Channelrhodopsin-2 gene transduced into retinal ganglion cells restores functional vision in genetically blind rats. Exp Eye Res 2010;90:429–36.
59. Jowett N, Kearney RE, Knox CJ, et al. Toward the bionic face: a novel neuroprosthetic device paradigm for facial reanimation consisting of neural blockade and functional electrical stimulation. Plast Reconstr Surg 2019;143:62e–76e.
60. Kanumuri VV, Ameen B, Jowett N, et al. PS 959. Optogenetic stimulation of the facial nerve in a murine model. Presented at Association for Research in Otolaryngology 42nd MidWinter Meeting. Baltimore, MD, February 9–13, 2019.
61. Guex AA, Hight AE, Narasimhan S, et al. Auditory brainstem stimulation with a conformable microfabricated array elicits responses with tonotopically organized components. Hear Res 2019;377:339–52.
62. Bloch J, Lacour SP, Courtine G. Electronic dura mater meddling in the central nervous system. JAMA Neurol 2017;74:470–5.
63. Chen X, Rogers JA, Lacour SP, et al. Materials chemistry in flexible electronics. Chem Soc Rev 2019;48:1431–3.
64. Hirsch A, Michaud HO, Gerratt AP, et al. Intrinsically stretchable biphasic (solid-liquid) thin metal films. Adv Mater 2016;28:4507–12.
65. Minev IR, Musienko P, Hirsch A, et al. Biomaterials. Electronic dura mater for long-term multimodal neural interfaces. Science 2015;347:159–63.
66. Guex AA, Vachicouras N, Hight AE, et al. Conducting polymer electrodes for auditory brainstem implants. J Mater Chem B 2015;3:5021–7.
67. Inaoka T, Shintaku H, Nakagawa T, et al. Piezoelectric materials mimic the function of the cochlear sensory epithelium. Proc Natl Acad Sci U S A 2011;108: 18390–5.

Printed and bound by CPI Group (UK) Ltd, Croydon, CR0 4YY

03/10/2024

01040482-0016